MUNCHAUSEN'S SYNDROME BY PROXY

MUNCHAUSEN'S SYNDROME BY PROXY

Current Issues in Assessment, Treatment and Research

Editors

Gwen Adshead & Deborah Brooke

Imperial College Press

Published by

Imperial College Press
57 Shelton Street
Covent Garden
London WC2H 9HE

Distributed by

World Scientific Publishing Co. Pte. Ltd.
P O Box 128, Farrer Road, Singapore 912805
USA office: Suite 1B, 1060 Main Street, River Edge, NJ 07661
UK office: 57 Shelton Street, Covent Garden, London WC2H 9HE

British Library Cataloguing-in-Publication Data
A catalogue record for this book is available from the British Library.

MUNCHAUSEN'S SYNDROME BY PROXY

ISBN 1-86094-134-6

Printed in Singapore.

Contents

List of Contributors

Introduction
Gwen Adshead, Honorary Senior Lecturer/Consultant in Forensic Psychotherapy. Broadmoor Hospital, St George's Hospital Medical School and Traumatic Stress Clinic, Middlesex Hospital. Deborah Brooke, Consultant Forensic Psychiatrist, Bracton Clinic, Bexley Hospital, Kent.

1 **A 20-Year Overview**
Arnon Bentovim, Consultant Child & Adolescent Psycho-Analyst & Family Therapist. London Child & Family Consultation Service.

2 **International Perspectives on Munchausen Syndrome by Proxy**
Rachel Brown, Associate Professor University School of Medicine, Macon, G. A. Marc Feldman, Chair for Clinical Services & Associate Professor, Department of Psychiatry, University of Alabama.

3 **Child Abuse Specific to the Medical System**
Jon Jureidini, Head, Department of Psychological Medicine, Women's & Children's Hospital, Adelaide. Terence Donald, Head, Child Protection Service, Women's & Children's Hospital, Adelaide.

4 **The Extraordinary Case of Mrs H.**
Estela Welldon, Consultant Psychiatrist, Portman Clinic and Honorary Senior Lecturer in Psychotherapy, University of London.

5 **Munchausen's Syndrome by Proxy: A Perspective from Primary Care**
Michael Bannon, Consultant Paediatrician, Northwick Park & St Marks NHS Trust, London. Yvonne Carter, Professor of General Practice & Primary Case, Queen Mary & Westfield College, London.

14 **Treatment and Outcome for Victims**
Ian Mitchell, Professor, Department of Paediatrics & Head of Paediatric Respirology. University of Calgary.

15 **Ethical and Public Policy Issues in the Management of Munchausen's Syndrome by Proxy**
Gwen Adshead, Honorary Senior Lecturer/Consultant in Forensic Psychotherapy. Broadmoor Hospital, St George's Hospital Medical School and Traumatic Stress Clinic, Middlesex Hospital.

16 **Current Challenges in the Management of Perpetrators**
Deborah Brooke, Consultant Forensic Psychiatrist, Bracton Clinic, Bexley Hospital, Kent. Gwen Adshead, Honorary Senior Lecturer/Consultant in Forensic Psychotherapy. Broadmoor Hospital, St George's Hospital Medical School and Traumatic Stress Clinic, Middlesex Hospital.

17 **New Directions in Research and Development**
Christopher Bools, Consultant Child, Adolescent and Family Psychiatrist, Child & Family Therapy Service, St Aldhelm's Hospital Frome.

Introduction

GWEN ADSHEAD

*Honorary Senior Lecturer/Consultant in Forensic Psychotherapy,
Broadmoor Hospital, St George's Hospital Medical School and
Traumatic Stress Clinic, Middlesex Hospital*

DEBORAH BROOKE

*Consultant Forensic Psychiatrist, Bracton Clinic,
Bexley Hospital, Kent*

INTRODUCTION

The aim of this book is to provide a multi-disciplinary and international perspective on current understanding of Munchausen's Syndrome by Proxy (MSBP). It may be helpful to start by thinking about the term itself, which as many of the contributors point out has given rise to considerable confusion. The confusion is compounded by the anxiety that the behaviour generates in all the services involved; especially when legal proceedings, either criminal or civil are underway. As several authors suggest, the confusion may arise because of the comparative lack of knowledge available about the origins of the behaviour. Some labels such as MSBP or Fictitious Illness by Proxy suggest a pathology in the perpetrator; other labels, such as Fictitious Illness Syndrome, suggest a problem in the child. The fact that there are at least two parties involved (the child and the perpetrator) makes choosing a single diagnostic label difficult. Because it is probably too soon to be able to come to a certain conclusion about nomenclature, we have deliberately left the authors to choose their own term.

It is indicative of the interest that this condition has attracted that so many different disciplines can claim to be involved. This book has arisen out of that collective experience. The contributors note the importance of multi-disciplinary working when managing MSBP cases, and we have been fortunate to have opinions from social work, paediatrics, law and psychiatry. We regretted that it was not possible to obtain a contribution from a nursing perspective, since the management of MSBP often fall heavily on paediatric nurses. Likewise, we were unable to include a chapter on the developmental effects of sustained or repeated fear on these children, growing up in such a hostile environment.

The other voice which is missing is that of the perpetrator. MSBP is a condition characterised by secrecy and first-hand stories from perpetrators, usually mothers, are rare. Lack of knowledge may reflect a difficulty which arises when the "problem" is a type of behaviour, which is not easily observed or detected, and involves deception by the potential patient. There is even some confusion about who is the patient in these cases. The lack of first hand accounts may be a result of the womens' own uncertainty about their actions and motives, and desire to deny actions which are highly stigmatised; especially in cultures where motherhood is idealised, but not supported.

As forensic psychiatrists, we regularly see offenders with histories of abuse, trauma and damage which are clearly related to their subsequent violence to themselves and others. There is still much to be learnt about the long-term influence of homes where violence occurs on a daily basis. The literature has established the high prevalences of abuse, deprivation and loss in MSBP perpetrators. Because most perpetrators are women, a further complication of the management of MSBP cases is the lack of services for women offenders, especially perpetrators of child abuse where the offender is dangerous only to members of the family circle. The needs and pathologies of the small number of male perpetrators are even less known. Effective intervention and prevention strategies will not be possible until the origins of these behaviours are understood, especially the contribution of early adverse experiences.

We are glad to have international contributors as well as an international perspective from Marc Feldman and Rachel Brown, demonstrating the pervasiveness of this behaviour across countries. We still do not know whether this behaviour is found in cultures other than Eurocentric ones. It is plausible to argue that social construction of both illness and motherhood are influential in the development of MSBP behaviour.

Many colleagues have helped us in our work and influenced our thinking: especially Gill Mezey and John Gunn. It was the courageous and pioneering work by Professor David Southall and Martin Samuels in the detection of MSBP that first interested us in this area of study, We are grateful to all the contributors who worked hard on this book; we would also like to express our real gratitute to Anne Kavanagh who has worked so hard to help us bring this book to fruition.

Gwen Adshead and Deborah Brooke, August 1999

"At the age of 24 she also was diagnosed as suffering from osteogenesis imperfecta, although she has fewer fractures than her mother."

A quote from a report prepared about a woman who had smothered her child repeatedly in hospital.

CHAPTER 1

A 20-Year Overview

ARNON BENTOVIM

Consultant Child & Adolescent Psychiatrist,
Psycho-Analyst & Family Therapist,
London Child & Family Consultation Service,
Honorary Consultant Psychiatrist Great Ormond Street and
the Tavistock Clinic

INTRODUCTION

Meadow introduced the term "Munchausen by Proxy" in 1977 and called it — "the hinterland of child abuse" (Meadow, 1977). Just over a year earlier, we had published a paper (Rogers *et al.*, 1976) from Great Ormond Street Hospital entitled, "Non-accidental poisoning: an extended syndrome of child abuse". A brief review of these two papers gives an indication of the way in which the current concept of Munchausen Syndrome by Proxy has developed, and also helps in the understanding of some of the related confusion and difficulty that has arisen.

NON-ACCIDENTAL POISONING

The term "non-accidental poisoning" adopted in the Great Ormond Street paper was in line with contemporary concepts of child abuse, which at the time included a broad spectrum of abusive behaviour, ranging from child murder through physical injury sustained by older children to the less obviously parentally inflicted child morbidity and mortality, resulting from non-accidental poisoning. We were able to point to papers by Lanski (1974) and Lanski and Erikson (1974) demonstrating that poisoning of a child had already been described. These papers also showed the way in which family pathology — in this case major marital conflict — may have played a role in the mother inducing coma as a way of dealing with conflict. A further series of poisoned children was described at Great Ormond Street, with substantial associated mortality. Our 1976 paper described a plan of action which was in line with management of child abuse at the time.

Psychiatric assessment of this series of cases indicated extreme parental ambivalence towards the child. There could be an alternation of blame and attack, with parents struggling with severe psychiatric disorders. There was a pattern of disturbed family relationships, with marital partners who remained peripheral to the over-close relationship between child and abusive parent. Hospital admission could be construed as a dysfunctional solution to marital conflict.

Treatment relied on the parents' acknowledgement of their responsibility for the poisoning act, and hence for their abnormal relationship with the child. Possible reunion followed appropriate therapeutic work with individuals and the family. We noted that two of the mothers when confronted with the fact that they were poisoning their children, themselves precipitated their own hospital admission. We understood these cases of non-accidental poisoning of children as a way for the parents to manage their own distress.

MUNCHAUSEN BY PROXY

This is where the link with Meadow's paper on Munchausen Syndrome by Proxy is formed. Meadow described two cases: the first, similar to our cases, in which a child was poisoned with salt; the second, where the mother provoked extensive investigation of the child over time. Meadow linked this child's case to "Munchausen Syndrome" (Asher, 1951).

Meadow noted that the behaviour of mothers' falsifying their children's medical symptoms had not previously been described. He questioned whether the degree of falsification was rare, or simply unrecognised. Meadow contrasted the behaviour of normal mothers of sick children on the ward, with the unusually pleasant and cooperative behaviour of the Munchausen mothers. They flourished in the ward, as if they belonged and thrived on the attention that the staff gave to them. They actively encouraged paediatricians to discover what the physical problem was. It was the fabricated stories that led Meadow to raise the question of Munchausen Syndrome, which classically describes individuals who travel widely for treatment, describing dramatic and fabricated symptoms, and who discharge themselves when discovered.

It is currently recognised that Munchausen by Proxy has been used as a term to encompass the *attribution* of an illness state to the child (through description of physical symptoms, or falsification of specimens, temperature charts, etc.), the *induction* of an illness state (through the actual administration of noxious substances), and the *maintenance* of an illness state (by direct interference with wounds or fractures).

Unfortunately, the term itself — Munchausen by Proxy — has given rise to considerable confusion, particularly at the time when Beverly Allit's poisoning of children in her care was described as a form of Munchausen by Proxy. We attempted to simplify matters (Gray and Bentovim, 1996) by using the term "Induced Illness Syndrome" to link with our earlier use of the term non-accidental poisoning. The problem is that terms like "Munchausen by Proxy" do not indicate clearly whether there is a problem affecting a child, or an adult, or a situation. Other terms have been introduced to describe this form of child maltreatment where the adult falsifies physical and/or psychological signs and/or symptoms in a victim causing the victim to be regarded as ill or impaired by others. The parent or care-giver as perpetrator is then seen as somebody who intentionally falsifies the history, signs or symptoms in a child to meet their own self-serving psychological needs. These include Factitious Illness by Proxy (Bools, 1996), and Paediatric Condition (Illness Impairment or Symptom Falsification), which apply to the child; and Factitious Disorder by Proxy, which applies to the adult (Ayoub and Alexander, 1998).

In my view, this difficulty in defining the entity is because in the beginning, non-accidental poisoning and Munchausen by Proxy were not seen clearly as variants of a particularly dangerous form of child abuse. Currently, there is no doubt that this is a serious and highly dangerous form of abusive action, and should be seen as a form of child abuse. Indeed, Meadow writing in his original paper writes "None can doubt that these two children were abused, but the acts of abuse were so different in quality, periodicity, and planning from the more usual non-accidental injury, of childhood that I am uneasy about classifying these sad cases as variants of non-accidental injury" (Meadow, 1977). Meadow's view is clearly different from this now.

FURTHER DEVELOPMENTS

Since the original paper was written in 1977, over the past 20 years, there has been quite an extraordinary growth in the recognition of the syndrome. This is not a syndrome which is rare, but seems to be basically unrecognised. When sets of case notes for parents and children are examined, they may reveal hundreds of admissions occurring (for a large sibship), where children may have been extensively investigated all over the country. Considerable slowness still occurs in recognising the role of parents, not as supporters of their children with disability, but as causing disability and benefiting from it.

There is of course the danger that parents will be accused of causing a child's state when physicians are bereft of ideas, and cannot understand the pattern of the child's illness. It can be an easy and dangerous way of physicians accusing parents of causing their child's illness, rather than being concerned about the possibility, and carefully planning how to make a diagnosis so that confrontation is based on sound evidence.

Case reports and studies have revealed the extraordinary range of ways in which parents can induce or fabricate illness states in their children. Controversially, this may even extend to the induction of psychiatric states in children. A variety of physical symptoms have been described: suffocation, recurrent apnoea and sudden infant death (Meadow, 1980; Southall *et al.*, 1997); Obstetric Factitious Disorders (Jureidini, 1993), and allergic forms (Warner and Hathaway, 1984).

Less information is available about the perpetrators, although there have now been follow-up studies of individual psychopathology (Bools *et al.*, 1994). Male perpetrators have also been described (Meadow, 1998). What the different manifestations seem to have in common is a type of deception, described by Rosenberg as a "web of deceit" (Rosenberg, 1987).

BROADER CONCEPTS AND TREATMENT

Munchausen by Proxy can be stretched as a notion, as evidenced in a paper by Schreier, where he describes repeated false allegations of sexual abuse (Schreier, 1996). Schreier suggests that this situation could be construed as "Munchausen by Proxy", arguing that if Munchausen by Proxy reflects the need to create a dependent and/or hostile relationship with powerful individuals, then different types of professionals may be involved, including law enforcement agents. Meadow describes a similar set of cases, and also construes them as a form of Munchausen by Proxy (Meadow, 1993). Meadow attempts to define a difference between those parents who develop a belief that their child has been sexually abused as a means of preventing contact in marital breakdown, from parents alleging sexual abuse of their child as a means of gaining special attention and support for themselves. Inevitably, attempting to make a diagnosis on the basis of the psychological intention of the parent becomes extremely difficult. However, this notion has been used in court cases where a parent is making an allegation that the other parent has abused the child, and professionals have labelled this as a case of Munchausen by Proxy. This gives an idea of the degree of confusion which can arise.

The provision of treatment remains limited. Throughout the literature, the emphasis is on description and understanding of the process, rather than application of treatment. Indeed, the emphasis on perceiving mothers as suffering from severe personality disorders can preclude the possibility of treatment. Within the child abuse field, generally, there is a division between those who feel there should be punishment for offending patients, and those who feel that such parents need treatment and understanding. Within the current offender field, there is a major commitment to treatment because it is recognised that punishment alone does not change individuals, or ensure that they will be safe from reenacting abusive patterns. In their review, Davies et al. (1998) describe how cases of Munchausen by Proxy are currently being managed through the child protection approach.

GREAT ORMOND STREET EXPERIENCE, 1977–1996

A way of exploring the last 20 years is to examine what has happened in our own practice at Great Ormond Street, looking at the developments from our original work on non-accidental poisoning to a recent work describing a series of 43 children from 37 families, diagnosed as inducing illness states in their children. A detailed account of this research has been published previously (Gray and Bentovim, 1996), and only a small part of it will be discussed here. Our consistent practice has been to regard Munchausen by Proxy as a form of child abuse. We have required that there be a clear diagnosis made through careful observation, and close interdisciplinary work between the paediatric team and the psychosocial team of social workers, psychiatrists, psychologists. The series of 41 children from 37 families were all diagnosed by our own team. The management team has included case conferencing, child protection procedures and has suggested appropriate treatment for the parents.

We identified four different categories of behaviour within the group. What was common to them all was an escalating gravity of presenting symptoms, and an early history of concern about the child. The four categories were:

(1) *Failure to thrive through the active withholding of food.*
There were ten children noted in this category. Mothers could be observed withholding food from their children, resulting in the children spending long periods in hospital.

(2) *Highly "allergic" children, who receive insufficient amounts of food.*
There were five children in this category. The children's behavioural difficulties were accounted for by allergy to various food stuffs. Parents shopped around from one doctor to another in search of yet another food stuff which could be blamed for causing problems. Children were often denied food on this basis, and only after hospital testing did it become clear that the child's state was exaggerated.

(3) *Parents who described worrying symptoms in their children.*
There were 15 children in this category. Parents claimed that their children had stopped breathing, were having fits, or were passing large amounts of urine.

(4) *Active administration of substances, or active interference with a child's medical treatment.*

There were 11 children in this category. Nursing charts and medical tests were interfered with. Children were given unprescribed medications, salt and laxatives. There were four deaths in this group, indicating the seriousness of the behaviour.

Family characteristics did not distinguish between the four groups. What was common to all of them was an early history and concern about the child's health, which encouraged a medicalisation of any subsequent difficulty. We felt that this perception of the child's life being under constant threat was a key factor in the presenting problem. There was a pattern of escalation of gravity of the presenting problems, especially where the parent believed that the medical attention offered was inadequate. However, continuing medical investigation and treatment reinforced the child's status as a sick child, albeit unintentionally.

What was striking was the highly positive presentation of the parents, who appeared to be the best parents, most devoted and least concerned with themselves. They often had considerable professional support. It was often difficult to get a history from the parents of any personal history of their own difficulties. On detailed investigation, however, half the mothers had a history of psychiatric symptoms, but had received little psychiatric help. A significant proportion of the mothers (35%) had histories of emotional privation and/or physical abuse. They had also experienced significant loss or bereavement. These families were characterised by mothers carrying heavy burdens. A high percentage of the fathers were peripheral or absent from the home, and 40% of the mothers described chronic and serious marital problems.

A review of the histories revealed that 60% of the parents had problems associated with parenting earlier in their parenting careers. What seemed to be common was an intolerance of normal assertive behaviour by their children. The Munchausen parents construed this behaviour in terms of an early illness state in the child. Mothers were observed to be intensely involved with their children, not allowing others to undertake the children's care.

Follow-up of this series of children which were identified between 1984 and 1991 (Gray, Bentovim and Milla, 1995) gives a striking insight into the failure of the professional community at large to understand that these children had been abused. It was an indication of our failure to have communicated this issue effectively. Perhaps at that time in the child protection field, we were too involved with the issue of child sexual abuse.

In our follow-up between four and eight years after that original series were diagnosed, we noted the incredible variety of responses from professionals all around the country who were involved with us in planning for the children's longer-term care. We saw professionals who colluded with vehement denial by parents that they could have been responsible for such abuse. At follow-up, 32 of the 41 children were placed with their abusive parents and 21 were doing poorly in the longer term. This indicates failure to take seriously the process by which a parent can induce an illness state in a child. Eleven of 21 parents did work therapeutically in the context of a proper care plan and have made good progress. Their children's health improved, and their need to use children as a means to gain help and support decreased.

A MODEL TO UNDERSTAND ILLNESS INDUCTION/MUNCHAUSEN BY PROXY

The process of illness induction is complex, involving interaction between characteristics of the child, early perceptions of them being ill and the beliefs of the parent. Early privation, stressful and traumatic effects were experienced by mothers and some fathers which led to the genesis of relationship difficulties and essentially an ambivalent attitude to their own child. This ambivalence manifested itself as a medicalisation of the difficult relationship, and the presentation of the child as "ill". Seeking help by proxy through the child being referred for medical help then became a legitimate mode of seeking help for themselves. Responses from the medical system results in a co-construction of the illness state, and a reinforcement of the child as having problems, with a concurrent setting aside of the parent's own history of deprivation or stress.

Relationships with children and parental capacity become idealised; ambivalence and grievance is felt towards a child who is believed to drain limited resources; and normal behaviour which is seen as overwhelming is set aside. Seeking medical assistance maintains an idealised perception of themselves as parents, avoiding actions of a physically abusive nature. It requires the child to be perceived as ill, and any clue that this may be seen through results in having to create an illness state to maintain the interest and involvement of the medical system. Finally, children are seen as objects requiring care, so that painful and dangerous actions can be justified.

Such individuals maintain their conviction about their child's illness with an intensity which bordered on the delusional, and the extraordinary splitting between thought and action maintains this "delusional" state. Schreier and Libow (1993) describe the intensely ambivalent relationships which develop between the parent and the physician as an aspect of self idealisation as rescuing parent, and the physician as both a saviour and failure as the illness is not cured.

A comprehensive narrative of an illness state evolves, leading the paediatrician to refer to a tertiary service for ever more investigations. It required skilled paediatric teams working with a psychosocial group to interpret and make sense of the symptoms and the family situation to make a diagnosis of the illness induction, clarify the nature of abusive actions, and take appropriate protective action.

Our own findings were that unless paediatricians and care professionals could work together to make a clear and accurate diagnosis, it was not possible to prevent the cycle of illness induction rolling on, with families moving on from one area of the health care system to another. Care alone is not enough, as without thorough ongoing treatment programmes which address the personal and family dimension, the process will continue to be maintained.

We have become aware that one needs to look outside this group of children who are diagnosed within hospital contexts, to the many children whose parents obtain a great deal of support from the health care system through the illness and state of invalidity of their children. We are beginning to see children with long-term physical states, cerebral palsy and asthma who presented as being far more disabled than their conditions would indicate. Situations occur where apparently compliant parents do not ensure that appropriate physiotherapy is applied, or where appropriate medication is not administered. This serves to maintain support for the parent through the illness state of their children. It is only by viewing these patterns as a form of abuse, as an example of significant harm where failure of adequate parenting means that the child's physical and emotional development is not maximised, that an appropriate programme of care and therapeutic work can be applied.

CONCLUSIONS

Review of our practice over 20 years indicates that our first instinct was correct and that children whose abuse is routed through the medical pathway should be regarded as suffering from abuse which is physical, emotional or sexual. Indeed, there is a considerable overlap. In our own series, there were concerns that 35% of siblings may have been abused.

It seems that the perception of the particular child as different resulted from an early problem involving medical care, which sensitised the parents to see this child as ill. The child's behaviour was perceived as challenging and defiant, but interpreted as being the result of a long-standing medical state, rather than deserving punishment or other forms of abuse. Although some perpetrators were fathers, the majority of perpetrators were women. Perhaps care afforded to mothers through the health system, whether in their own childhood, during pregnancy and early in their children's lives, may play a part in them seeing the medical system as offering non-possessive warmth, accurate empathy and uncritical concern. Given the levels of privation, loss and abuse these mothers had experienced, the medical system may well be seen as a haven of support and care. So the seed may be sown for this group of children to experience their parents' ambivalence through the induction of an illness state, and an ever deepening conviction that what is required is medical care for that child, with secondary support for the parent being the hidden gain.

Any form of abusive behaviour towards a child requires protection for the child, support for the family, and a therapeutic programme to tackle the abusive pattern in the parent. If it proves impossible to engage or work with the parent and help them acknowledge their abusive act, then the child deserves and requires long-term care in a safe context. At follow-up, all children placed in alternative contexts to their own parents thrived and did well, whereas children placed with their parents were more likely to do poorly. There were deaths, and there was only improvement when there was a concerted therapeutic programme of work for parents and a care plan for the benefit and safety of the children.

The next 20 years of study ought to focus on the development of therapeutic services which can work preventatively with those deprived and abused parents who have sick infants. Preventative work can be successful in ensuring that the children develop safely in homes where there are high risks. This group of children demonstrates the need to continue and intensify preventative intervention.

The boundaries of Munchausen by Proxy have not been set in this 20-year period, and it is evident that parents can seek attention, care and support for themselves through their children in many ways. In my view, we need to understand the processes which lead parents to seek such attention through medical channels, or recognise such events accurately, and to intervene so as to treat and prevent them. We will have helped many children and families to live healthier lives if we are successful!

REFERENCES

Asher, R. (1951). Munchausen's Syndrome. *Lancet* **1**: 339–341.

Ayoub, C. C., Alexander, R. (1988). Definitial issues in Munchausen by Proxy. *American Professional Society of the Abuse of Children Adviser* **11**: 7–10.

Bools *et al.* (1994). Munchausen's Syndrome by Proxy. A study of psychopathology. *Child Abuse Negl.* **18**: 773–788.

Bools *et al.* (1996). Factitious illness by proxy (Munchausen's Syndrome by Proxy). *Br. J. Psychiat.* **169**: 268–275.

Davies, P., McClure, Rolff, K., Chessman, N., Pearson, S., Sibert, J. R., Meadow, R. (1998). Procedures, placement and risks of further abuse after Munchausen

Syndrome by Proxy, non-accidental poisoning, and non-accidental suffocation. *Arch. Dis. Child.* **78**: 217–221.

Gray, J., Bentovim, A., Milla, P. (1995). The treatment of children and their families where induced illness has been identified. *Trust betrayed? Munchausen Syndrome by Proxy, Interagency Child Protection and Partnership with Families*, edited by J. Horwath and B. Lawson. National Children's Bureau.

Gray, J., Bentovim, A. (1996). Illness induction syndrome: paper 1 — a series of 41 children from 37 families identified at the Great Ormond Street Hospital for Children NHS Trust. *Child Abuse Negl.* **20**: 655–673.

Jureidini, J. (1993). Obstetric Factitious Disorder and Munchausen Syndrome by Proxy. *Nerv. Ment. Dis.* **181(2)**: 135–137.

Lanski, L. L. (1974). An unusual case of childhood chloral hydrate poisoning. *Am. J. Dis. Child.* **127**: 275–276.

Lanski, S. B., Erikson, H. M. (1974). Prevention of child murder. A case report. *J. Am. Acad. Child. Psychiat.* **13**: 691–698.

Meadow, R. (1977). Munchausen Syndrome by Proxy — the hinterland of child abuse. *Lancet* **2**: 343–357.

Meadow, R. (1990). Suffocation, recurrent apnoea and sudden infant death. *The J. Paediatr.* **117**: 351–357.

Meadow, R. (1993). False allegations of abuse and Munchausen Syndrome by Proxy. *Arch. Dis. Child.* **68**: 444–447.

Meadow, R. (1998). Male perpetrators of Munchausen by Proxy. *Arch. Dis. Child.* **78**: 380–386.

Rogers, D., Trip, J., Bentovim, A., Robinson, A., Berry, D., Goulding, R. (1976). Non accidental poisoning: An extended syndrome of child abuse. *Br. Med. J.* **1**: 793–796.

Rosenberg, D. (1987). Web of Deceit: A literature review of Munchausen by Proxy. *Child Abuse Negl.* **11**: 547–563.

Schreier, H. A., Libow, J. A. (1993). *Hurting for Love. Munchausen by Proxy Syndrome* (Guilford Books, New York).

Schreier, H. A. (1996). Repeated false allegations of sexual abuse presenting to sheriffs: When is it Munchausen by Proxy? *Child Abuse Negl.* **20**: 985–991.

Southall, D., Plunkett, C., Banks, M., Falcov, A., Samuels, M. (1997). Covert video recordings of life threatening child abuse: Lessons for child protection. *Paediatrics* **160**: 735–760.

Warner, J. O., Hathaway, M. J. (1984). Allergic form of Meadow's syndrome (Munchausen by Proxy). *Arch. Dis. Child.* **59**: 151–156.

CHAPTER 2

International Perspectives on Munchausen Syndrome by Proxy

RACHEL M. A. BROWN, M. B., B. S.,
M. PHIL., M. R. C. Psych.
Associate Professor,
Mercer University School of Medicine,
Macon, Georgia

MARC D. FELDMAN, M. D.
Vice Chair for Clinical Services & Associate Professor,
Department of Psychiatry,
University of Alabama at Birmingham,
Birmingham, Alabama

INTRODUCTION

With relatively few exceptions, the literature about Munchausen Syndrome by Proxy (MSBP) has been written by professionals working in the United States, the United Kingdom, Canada, Australia, and New Zealand. Not surprisingly, these reviews, reports, and analyses focus on the presentation and management of the phenomenon as it has arisen in those countries. In this chapter, we aim to extend the discussion beyond these geographic borders by reviewing the literature that has emerged from other countries. We will also offer preliminary thoughts about the cross-cultural issues that may be relevant in understanding, investigating, and managing MSBP.

As far as we know, this chapter represents the first published effort to perform such a review. Daunting roadblocks have appeared along the way and we will acknowledge them now. First, lacking access to a polyglot, we were able to elicit details only from papers published in English or containing English abstracts. In some cases, we were left to infer the relevance of an article based only on the translation of a title. However, we have not included information that represented mere speculation or supposition. Second, MSBP is, even within the countries noted above, little known compared with most other forms of abuse. Ostfeld and Feldman (1996) found in a U.S. survey that 89% of the child–psychiatrist respondents had heard of MSBP but only 42% of social workers had. The same authors noted that the availability of articles about MSBP varies markedly among the professional disciplines involved in the assessment and care of children and families, and the working definitions of MSBP sometimes differ (Meadow, 1995; Jones, 1996). Yet another variable affecting knowledge level is the particular setting in which clinicians practice; Kaufman et al. (1989), for example, found that clinicians in intensive medical settings such as hospitals were three times as likely to be aware of MSBP as those who practiced in the community. These considerations are relevant to the task of this chapter because MSBP is undoubtedly even less well-known, at least by name, in countries in which the professional literature is limited in scope, distribution, and accessibility. The relatively few published examples of MSBP in other cultures, then, may reflect limited awareness of the existence and definition of this form of abuse rather than actual incidence and prevalence. Third, even the scattered reports that do appear from developing countries may not be representative of the phenomenology of MSBP in those parts of the world. Individuals who choose to write and publish case reports are a self-selected group whose backgrounds and training may differ from those of their colleagues. Similarly, the international articles that do exist may have been reported only because they approximate cases which are already available in the published literature. Finally, our hypotheses and conclusions are necessarily constrained by the limits of our knowledge about the rates, type, and meaning of abuse and neglect across cultures and ethnic groups (Garbarino and Ebata, 1983; Amirali et al., 1998). Rather than offer the "final word" on the subject of international perspectives on MSBP, we hope instead to facilitate ongoing discussion.

CROSS-CULTURAL INFLUENCES ON RATES OF MSBP

Garbarino and Ebata (1983) note that cultural and ethnic differences in rates of abuse and neglect have received little formal study. Their review, however, led them to form tentative conclusions that may be useful in considering international aspects of MSBP. They point out that, within the United States, there is greater variability *within* particular subcultures than *between* subcultures. If this general observation holds true for MSBP, we might expect rather small differences among countries. However, Garbarino and Ebata also suggest that there are factors within each society and subculture, such as values, practices, and biological predisposition — that appear to render its children particularly vulnerable or resistant to particular forms of child maltreatment. If so, we can only speculate about the ways in which such vulnerabilities or resistances may impact the frequency and manifestations of MSBP maltreatment. Garbarino and Ebata note that the *form*, rather than the *rate* of child abuse or neglect, may be most influenced by cultural factors. They cite the example of dual mother–child suicide-homicide, a phenomenon that is relatively common in Japan but rare in other countries. Again, if this observation applies to MSBP as well, then we may expect that MSBP will arise much more frequently in the medicalised atmospheres of Western countries. While we cannot reliably determine the cross-cultural rates of MSBP and must continually bear in mind the caveats that opened this chapter, we can offer statements about the form it takes based upon our review of the available case reports.

THE EVOLUTION OF KNOWLEDGE

The first U.S. reports of MSBP did not appear until some 30 years after American medicine began to focus on the maltreatment of children (Caffey, 1946). To hypothesise about the likely path of international awareness and conceptualisations of MSBP, it is helpful first to consider the "developmental history" of MSBP in the West.

Reports of single cases or small series (Rogers *et al.*, 1976; Meadow, 1977) began to appear in the late seventies. Over time, larger series of cases explicitly identified as MSBP were published (e.g., Gray and Bentovim,

1996). Review articles emerged about ten years after the first reports (e.g., Rosenberg, 1987; Byard and Beal, 1993; Eminson and Postlethwaite, 1992), and there was a gradual increase in articles examining details such as the frequency of the condition among siblings (Lee, 1979; Bools *et al.*, 1992) and the presence of adult factitious disorders among some MSBP perpetrators (Janofsky, 1986; Feldman *et al.*, 1997; Meadow, 1999). With increasing awareness and detection, selected authors attempted to elucidate the prevalence of MSBP within particular referred populations, such as children presenting with apnea (0.27% — Light and Sheridan, 1989), allergy (5% — Warner and Hathaway, 1984), asthma (1% — Godding and Kruth, 1981), apparent life-threatening episodes (1.5% — Rahilly, 1991), and life-threatening episodes treated with cardiopulmonary resuscitation (over 9% among children in whom final diagnoses were established — Samuels *et al.*, 1993). There have even been recent attempts at epidemiology within the British Isles (McClure *et al.*, 1996; Davis *et al.*, 1998). During the late 1980s and 1990s, single case reports have been increasingly limited to notably unusual presentations, such as fathers (Makar and Squier, 1990; Porter *et al.*, 1994) or nurses as perpetrators (Repper, 1995; Yorker, 1996), or fetuses (Pickford *et al.*, 1988; Jureidini, 1993) or adults as victims (Smith and Ardern, 1989; Sigal *et al.*, 1986, 1991; Ben-Chetrit and Melmed, 1998). At the same time, controversies such as the legal and ethical issues in covert video surveillance (CVS) have generated a great deal of debate, particularly in the United States and Britain (The Lancet, 1994; Yorker, 1995; Shinebourne, 1996). The phenomenon is now routinely portrayed in professional newspapers (Clinical Psychiatry News, 1993) and the popular press (The Guardian, 1993). "True crime" books involving MSBP have been published in increasing numbers (Wright, 1984; Egginton, 1989; Elkind, 1990; Davies, 1993; Cavenaugh, 1995; Olsen, 1995; Firstman and Talan, 1997). Within the past few years, there have been burgeoning efforts to delimit use of the term, since usage has appeared injudicious at times (e.g., Meadow, 1995) and misdiagnoses have been reported (Meadow, 1993; Rand and Feldman, 1999). Chapters on MSBP in books on abuse predate books devoted entirely to MSBP (Schreier and Libow, 1993b; Levin and Sheridan, 1996; Parnell and Day, 1997; Artingstall, 1998; Eminson and Postlethwaite, 1999), such as this one. The first such book, *Hurting for Love*, appeared in 1993, almost 20 years after Meadow's (1977) seminal report of the condition.

This pattern would be expected to repeat itself in countries in which awareness of MSBP has developed more recently. The first report of MSBP we have seen from outside the United States, United Kingdom, Canada, Australia, or New Zealand is from Israel (Shnaps *et al.*, 1981). It appeared in *Pediatrics*, a journal published in English and, like other English-language reports, probably reflects a common professional culture across countries. A number of articles in English from other parts of the world and among diverse medical specialties have appeared subsequently (see Table 1).

As Table 1 indicates, foreign language reports of MSBP — in French (Douchain *et al.*, 1987; DeToni *et al.*, 1987; Ginies *et al.*, 1989), Italian (Caruso *et al.*, 1989), Spanish (Jiminez Hernandez *et al.*, 1987; Reig del Moral *et al.*, 1986; Palomeque *et al.*, 1986), and Dutch (Feenstra *et al.*, 1988; Hulstijn-Dirkmaat *et al.*, 1987) — began to appear in the European literature in the mid-to-late eighties. Since then, reports have come from South and Central America (Loredo-Abdala *et al.*, 1991 [Mexico]; Chantada *et al.*, 1994 [Argentina]; Guiraldes *et al.*, 1995 [Chile]) and from other parts of Europe, including Poland (Ksiazyk *et al.*, 1990), Belgium (Adriaensens and Eggermont, 1991), Germany (Guenter and Boos, 1994; Krupinski *et al.*, 1995; Marcus *et al.*, 1995a, 1995b), Scandinavia (Carlson *et al.*, 1994; Hertz *et al.*, 1993), Turkey (Senocak *et al.*, 1995), and the former Czechoslovakia (Vondrak *et al.*, 1995) and Yugoslavia (Martinovic, 1995). Articles presenting unusual cases (Sigal *et al.*, 1986, 1991) and discussing local legal issues (Sigal *et al.*, 1990) have emerged from Israel. Over the last few years, the first reports have come from Africa (Ifere *et al.*, 1993; Oyelami *et al.*, 1994), Saudi Arabia (Al-Jumaah *et al.*, 1993), the Indian subcontinent (Bhatia, 1990; Perera *et al.*, 1995), and the Far East (Lim *et al.*, 1991; Honjo, 1996). These papers are in English, probably reflecting the fact that English is, in many countries, the *lingua franca* of tertiary education. We have not uncovered any published reports from China or the former Soviet Union, but our access to this literature is limited.

In summary, published reports of MSBP have come from a broad array of countries all over the world. Table 1 summarises 53 reports involving more than 110 cases outside the United States, United Kingdom, Canada,

Table 1.   International published reports of MSBP.[1]

Authors and Date	Country	Language	No. of Cases	Age, Sex of Victim (s)	Perpetrator	Nature of MBP
Douchain, 1987	France?	French	1	NA[2]	NA	Factitious urinary lithiasis
Ginies et al., 1989	France	French	1	4.5 years, M[3]	Mother	Chronic barbiturate intoxication leading to enteral feeding, ileostomy and total parenteral nutrition
Ginies et al., 1996	France	French	1	Infant, F	NA	NA
Bertheir and Oriot, 1996	France?	French	1	NA, F	Mother	NA
Bouden et al., 1996	France	French	NA	NA	NA	NA
Krebs et al., 1996	France	French	1	Adult, M	Wife of victim	Repeated tranquilizer injection leading to coma
Vouzemoix, 1995	Switzerland?	French	1	NA, M	Mother	NA
Caruso et al., 1989	Italy	Italian	1	12 years, M	Mother	Administration of glibenclamide leading to hypoglycemia and subtotal pancreatectomy
DeToni et al., 1987	Italy	Italian	1	NA	NA	NA

Table 1. *(Continued)*

Authors and Date	Country	Language	No. of Cases	Age, Sex of Victim (s)	Perpetrator	Nature of MBP
Mengarda *et al.*, 1995	Italy	Italian	1	Infant, NA	Parent (unspecified)	Factitious vomiting and failure to thrive
Baracchini *et al.*, 1995	Italy	Italian	2	NA	NA	NA
D'Avanzo *et al.*, 1995	Italy	English	1	4.5 years, M	Mother	Furosemide poisoning leading to misdiagnosis of Bartter syndrome
Loredo-Abdala *et al.*, 1991	Mexico	Spanish	2	NA, F NA, M	NA	NA
Chantada *et al.*, 1994	Argentina	English	4	Four "older children," 3 F, 1 M	NA	Factitious fever of unknown origin in all cases
Guiraldes *et al.*, 1995	Chile	Spanish	3	1) 9 years, F 2) 13 years, F 3) 14 years, F (unrelated)	Mother in 2 cases, father in 1	Recurrent hematemesis in 2 cases, melena in 1
Ksiazyk *et al.*, 1990	Poland	Polish	1	> 6 years, F	NA	Potassium chloride added to faeces, natrium hydrocarbonate added to urine, furosemide administered; symptoms included polyuria, hyponatremia, hypokalemia

Table 1. (Continued)

Authors and Date	Country	Language	No. of Cases	Age, Sex of Victim (s)	Perpetrator	Nature of MBP
Shnaps et al., 1981	Israel	English	1	18 months, F	Mother	Recurrent chlorpromazine poisoning
Roth, 1990	Israel	English	4	NA	NA	"Mild" MBP in all cases
Sigal et al., 1986, 1991	Israel	English	3	1) Adult, F 2) Adult, F 3) Adult, M (unrelated)	Husband of victim 1	Administration of hypnotics and injection of gasoline or turpentine
Ben-Chetrit and Melmed, 1998	Israel	English	1	73 years, F	Daughter?	Injection of insulin to cause hypoglycemia
Al-Jumaah et al., 1993	Saudi Arabia	English	1	15 months, F	Mother	Applications of an alkaline detergent to cause ulcers to oropharynx
Bhatia, 1990	India	English	1	Adolescent, M	Mother	Factitious hematuria (blood added to urine)
Somani, 1998	India	English	1	28 years, M	Wife	Burning of facial skin with acid
Reig del Moral et al., 1986	Spain?	Spanish	4	1) 2 years, NA 2) 12 months, NA 3) > 6 years, F 4) NA (siblings)	Mother	NA

Table 1. *(Continued)*

Authors and Date	Country	Language	No. of Cases	Age, Sex of Victim (s)	Perpetrator	Nature of MBP
Palomeque *et al.*, 1986	Spain	Spanish	1	9 years, F	Mother	Imipramine poisoning leading to neurological symptoms and acute intermittent porphyria diagnosis
Jiminez Hernandez *et al.*, 1987	Spain	Spanish	NA	NA	NA	NA
Jiminez Hernandez and Figuerido-Poulin, 1996	Spain	Spanish	20 (cases accumulated from Spanish literature)	NA (20 separate families)	Mother in all cases	Drug intoxication in 13 cases; others NA
Gomez de Terreros *et al.*, 1996	Spain	Spanish	1	10 months, NA	Mother	Fed foreign objects
Fernandez-Jaen *et al.*, 1998	Spain	English	1	8 years, M	Mother	Seizures induced by clomipramine poisoning in setting of genuine seizure disorder
Lesnik Oberstein, 1986	Netherlands	Dutch	1	3 years, F	Mother	NA

Table 1. (Continued)

Authors and Date	Country	Language	No. of Cases	Age, Sex of Victim (s)	Perpetrator	Nature of MBP
Hulstijn-Dirkmaat et al., 1987	Netherlands	Dutch	NA	NA	NA	NA
Feenstra et al., 1988	Netherlands	Dutch?	1	1 year, F	Grandmother (foster mother)	Alum injected into parotid gland
Prakken et al., 1991	Netherlands	Dutch	1	11 years, M	Father	Cooked meat added to urine; false report of hematuria and abdominal pain
de Ridder et al., 1998	Netherlands	Dutch	2	1) 4 years, F 2) Approx. 1 year, M	Mother in both cases	Fabrication and falsification to cause 1) Diarrhoea, vomiting, and temperature elevation 2) Cyanosis and tachycardia
Hoorntje et al., 1999	Netherlands	Dutch	1	14 months, M	Mother	Repeated cyanosis and loss of consciousness caused by strangulation
Adriaenssens and Eggermont, 1991	Belgium	Dutch	>1	NA	Mother	Administration of tranquilizers

Table 1. *(Continued)*

Authors and Date	Country	Language	No. of Cases	Age, Sex of Victim (s)	Perpetrator	Nature of MBP
Godding and Kruth, 1991	Belgium	English	17 families	4–12 years, 12 M, 5 F	Mother in 13 cases, father in 1 case, grandmother in 2 cases, both parents in 1 case	Aggravation of asthma in 10; exaggerated symptoms of asthma in 7
Marcus et al., 1995a	Germany	English	4	1) 4.5 years, M 2) 3 years, F 3) 6 years, F 4) 9 years, F	1) Mother 2) Mother 3) Mother 4) Mother	1) Laxative ingestion leading to gastrointestinal dysfunction 2) False sexual abuse report 3) Factitious melena, allergy, seizures, blurred vision, and false sexual abuse report 4) Factitious seizures
Marcus et al., 1995b	Germany	English	1	11 years, M	Mother	Benzodiazepine administration leading to psychotic symptoms
Gunter and Boos, 1994	Germany	German	1	NA, F	20-year-old female	"Induced borderline psychosis"
Krupinski et al., 1995	Germany	German	1	12 years, M	Mother	Unwarranted confinement to wheelchair and implantation of pacemaker

Table 1. *(Continued)*

Authors and Date	Country	Language	No. of Cases	Age, Sex of Victim (s)	Perpetrator	Nature of MBP
Kaufman-Walther and Laederach-Hoffmann, 1997	Switzerland	German	1	NA, M	Mother	NA
Vondrak et al., 1995	Former Czechoslovakia	Serbo-Croat?	1	NA	NA	Factitious hematuria leading to renal biopsy
Martinovic, 1995	Former Yugoslavia	English	4	1) 5 years, M 2) 7 years, M 3) 13 years, F 4) 14 years, F (unrelated)	1) Mother 2) Mother 3) Mother 4) Father	Fictitious epilepsy in all cases
Carlson et al., 1994	Sweden	English	1	6 years, M	Mother	Administration of laxative (Glauber's salt) leading to severe diarrhoea
Hertz et al., 1995	Norway	Norwegian?	2	NA (siblings)	NA	NA
Moszkowicz and Bjørnholm, 1998	Denmark	English	1	2 years, M	Mother	Restriction of food and overfeeding of water leading to nonorganic failure to thrive

Table 1. *(Continued)*

Authors and Date	Country	Language	No. of Cases	Age, Sex of Victim (s)	Perpetrator	Nature of MBP
Ifere *et al.*, 1993	Nigeria	English	1	11 years, M	Mother	False reports of fever of unknown origin, asthma, tuberculosis, carditis, urinary dysfunction, diabetes mellitus
Oyelami *et al.*, 1994	Nigeria	English	2	1) 2.5 years, M 2) 4–5 years, F (siblings)	Mother	Factitious bleeding, dyspnea, cough, fever, fainting
Lim *et al.*, 1991	Singapore	English	1	15 months, M	Mother	False reports, including frequent gastroenteritis and "viral fever"
Senocak *et al.*, 1995	Turkey	English	1	2 years, M	Father's second wife (not child's mother)	Stones inserted into urethra
Perera *et al.*, 1995	Sri Lanka	English	1	8 months, F	Mother	False reports of hematemesis, hematochezia, and convulsions
Honjo, 1996	Japan	English	1	25 months, F	Mother	Underfeeding with false reports of overeating

[1]Excludes United States, United Kingdom, Australia, New Zealand, and Canada

[2]NA = information not available to authors

[3]M = male; F = female

Australia, and New Zealand. Meadow (personal communication, September 1997) indicates that, beyond cases that have appeared in print, he has heard of cases from every continent, all the countries of Western Europe, almost every country in Eastern Europe, the Arab countries of the Middle East, and the Far East.

CROSS-CULTURAL PRESENTATIONS OF MSBP

It is striking to note that the signs and symptoms feigned or induced appear, with an exception to be noted, largely consistent across the world. Although possible reporting bias means we must apply this conclusion with caution, it accords with a comment made by Meadow (personal communication, September 1997): "To me it seems that the type of abuse is similar in all countries.... The stories from the perpetrating mothers and their actions seem to be the same regardless of the geography or the culture." Common presentations include fabricated or induced bleeding (particularly urinary or gastrointestinal), other gastrointestinal symptoms, surreptitious administration of harmful substances and foreign objects, false reports of seizures, and spurious claims of fever and failure to thrive. Oddly, however, there are almost no cases in the table involving apnea, which has historically been among the most commonly reported ailments (Rosenberg, 1987). Differentiation of forcible respiratory arrest from spontaneous apnea and sudden infant death syndrome (SIDS) continues to be a complex undertaking (Firstman and Talan, 1997), and it is possible that such cases have occurred worldwide but have eluded detection. As in English-speaking industrialised countries, however, feigned or induced psychological and behavioral variants of MSBP are rarely reported, though the phenomenon itself is not necessarily rare.

The age of the victims in the table is similar to that of reported cases — almost always pre-pubertal — with perpetrators being the mothers in most cases in which the perpetrator is known. The father is the perpetrator in four cases (Guiraldes *et al.*, 1995; Prakken *et al.*, 1991; Martinovic, 1995; Godding and Kruth, 1991), another family member is culpable in six cases (Krebs *et al.*, 1996; Sigal *et al.*, 1986, 1991; Feenstra *et al.*, 1988; Godding and Kruth, 1991; Senocak *et al.*, 1995), both parents are involved in one case (Godding and Kruth, 1991), and the victim and assailant are unrelated in two cases (Sigal *et al.*, 1991). The presence of the syndrome in more than one child of the same family is reported in several instances (e.g., Reig del Moral *et al.*, 1986; Hertz *et al.*, 1995; Oyelami *et al.*, 1994), reinforcing the concept of serial or multi-victim MSBP. When detailed case descriptions were available to us, they were very similar to those with which the English-speaking audience is familiar: the repeated presentation of children with a variety of symptoms, multiple fruitless medical investigations, and the repeated denial by the perpetrator of her role in the child's plight even when the evidence is incontrovertible (Feldman, 1994).

Just as Rosenberg's 1987 article (Rosenberg, 1987) heralded efforts to synthesise the English-language MSBP literature, review articles have now appeared in other languages as well. They include Dutch (Koopman and Feenstra, 1988), German (Freyberger and Freyberger, 1997), Spanish (Jimenez Hernandez and Figuerido-Poulain, 1996), Hebrew (Lerner and Witztum, 1998) and French (Bouden *et al.*, 1996; Bocquet *et al.*, 1997). Consolidations of the literature have also appeared in English from Israel (Sigal *et al.*, 1989) and Denmark (Skau and Mouridsen, 1995). Large case series are missing, however, from foreign language reports, as is much discussion of rare or previously-unknown variants of MSBP or specific diagnostic, ethical, or legal controversies. As we have said, Israel is probably a special case. We failed to uncover any attempts to examine the relative incidence and prevalence of this form of abuse in different countries, though there are suggestions that it is probably underreported (Jimenez Hernandez and Figureido-Poulain, 1996) and that it may be increasing in frequency (Oyelami *et al.*, 1994). This surfeit of epidemiologic studies is not surprising since, as noted, it is only recently that serious efforts at community-based surveys have emerged in the United Kingdom (McClure *et al.*, 1996), where the condition was first described.

The report by McClure *et al.* (1996) merits additional attention as we seek to establish an international perspective on MSBP. This article describes a seven-fold difference in reported incidence by region even within a country as geographically small as England. Perhaps, mirroring the observation of Garbarino and Ebata (1983), MSBP — like other forms of abuse — varies as much (or more) *within* as *among* cultures. As McClure *et al.* (1996) speculate, there are several possible reasons for the regional variations in reports and these may be applicable across countries. First, there may, of course, be true differences in frequency from place to place. Second, the educational backgrounds and professional milieu of paediatricians and others may affect awareness. Reports of MSBP arise more frequently in countries which use English in sharing professional findings, for instance. However, the absence of reports from South Africa mitigates against this point. Third, the potential for diagnosing MSBP may be reduced in settings with large numbers of paediatricians since "doctor shopping" can go undetected more easily. If this speculation is true, then countries with very few physicians might be expected to have much higher rates of diagnosed MSBP, especially if the existing physicians were interested in the condition. Finally, there are the potential problems of lack of recognition of and unwillingness to report MSBP in certain societies and subcultures. If we assume that countries with high rates of poverty, malnutrition, and infant and child mortality, and with poor health and social services systems, have been slower to focus on child abuse as a public health concern, then we must assume that they will be even slower to recognise MSBP per se. After all, as described earlier, the lag was around 30 years in the United Kingdom and United States.

We are aware of no other books devoted to MSBP except in English. If we are correct in our assumption that the recognition of the phenomenon may take a similar course in each country, we would not have expected them to have appeared yet. Lacking access to the periodicals favored by the citizens in other countries, we do not know whether the condition has emerged from the professional literature into the public eye, though we would predict that such mass media presentations would be infrequent to date.

CROSS-CULTURAL PERSPECTIVES ON ETIOLOGY

It is likely that the professional education and experiences of authors and the prevailing theoretical paradigms within which they work have shaped the hypotheses advanced to account for MSBP. Hypotheses in the international literature are largely of three types: conventional diagnoses that are viewed tacitly as "etiologic" (Shnaps *et al.*, 1981); psychodynamic theories of varying complexity (Kennedy and Coombe, 1995; Schreier and Libow, 1993); or broader syntheses of the interactions among mother, father, child, and the medical system (Gray and Bentovim, 1992).

The first type of approach is reflected in references from as far afield as Scandinavia and Africa. These papers discuss either diagnosable mental illness in the mother (Shnaps *et al.*, 1981), or general parental psychopathology (Marcus *et al.*, 1995a, 1995b; Sigal *et al.*, 1995; Skau and Mouridsen, 1995; Perera *et al.*, 1995; Ifere *et al.*, 1993; Carlson *et al.*, 1994; Jiminez Hernandez and Figuerido-Poulain, 1996; Honjo, 1996; Godding and Kruth, 1991). The second type is particularly evident in the French literature, which often appears to focus on psychodynamic formulations of maternal pathology (Krebs *et al.*, 1996; Bouden *et al.*, 1996), although it is possible that this orientation is idiosyncratic to the authors rather than culturally determined. The third type, mother–child interaction difficulties and family dynamics, are commonly discussed in other papers (Martinovic, 1995; Sigal *et al.*, 1989; Shnaps *et al.*, 1981; Guiraldes *et al.*, 1995; Skau and Mouridsen, 1995; Godding and Kruth, 1991; Perera *et al.*, 1995; Ifere *et al.*, 1993), and well-illustrated by the report by Sigal *et al.* (1989) which refers to the "triad of mother, child and medicine." In this context, three authors view marital issues as specifically etiologic in the cases they discuss. In Solami's (1998) paper, a woman repeatedly burned her unconscious husband's cheek with acid to frighten him and dissuade him from drinking. Senocak *et al.* (1995) felt that the motivation of the abusive stepmother, who inserted pebbles into a boy's urethra, was revenge on her bigamous husband, his second wife, and the child the two had together. Oyelami *et al.* (1994) cite the mother's wish to bankrupt her husband in order to prevent a second polygamous marriage as one factor in a case from West Africa. Issues of bigamy are obviously rare in Western medical practice. Also, in all three cases a diagnosis of "malingering by proxy" (Feldman *et al.*, 1997) may be more appropriate than MSBP since the goal appears to have been extrinsic to assumption of the sick role by proxy.

The possibility that modern medicine itself may be etiologic in MSBP is a challenging one. Most authors have seen physicians as the unwitting victims of the perpetrating mothers, who betray them and their children in the service of meeting their own needs. Donald and Jureidini (1996), however, have suggested that medical practice itself contributes to the condition. They believe that "...poor history taking is central to its etiology... [and] medical interest and active participation is the crucial factor in the maintenance of the syndrome." Although they stop short of declaring modern medicine as etiologic, Oyelami et al. (1994) do view the influence of Western culture as contributing centrally to the emergence of MSBP in Nigeria. They write, "...as our society continues to imbibe Western habits, rightly or wrongly, this rather common form of child abuse in developed countries may be causing diagnostic puzzles for medical practitioners in developing countries." Interestingly, however, they also comment on the role that traditional healers may have played in the case they report — healers zealously offer "remedies" with potential morbidity of their own, and they do not regularly share information and coordinate efforts with others in the community who may also be caring for the child.

MANAGEMENT

Within the English-language Western literature, there is a reasonable consensus on how MSBP is best detected and initially managed (Meadow, 1985; Ostfeld and Feldman, 1996), and many of the foreign language reports from Western countries appear to be in agreement. The commonest error in the diagnostic process — namely, failure to consider MSBP in the differential (Mitchell et al., 1993) — appears to occur everywhere. There are repeated exhortations in the international literature to greater awareness (e.g., Skau and Mouridsen, 1995; Carlson et al., 1994; Krebs et al., 1996; Perera et al., 1995; Loredo-Abdala et al., 1991). If, as Mitchell et al. (1993) suggest, the ability to recognise and manage MSBP improves with experience, we should expect increasing numbers of cases to be reported worldwide over time.

Undoubtedly, the thorough acquisition of information is the core of good medicine no matter where it is practiced. However, the specifics of obtaining this information may well differ by culture. For example, Meadow (1985), practicing in the United Kingdom, has advocated that clinicians make unannounced visits to the family's home to inspect the environment, or that they perform unauthorized searches of belongings, both of which would probably be illegal in the United States. Similarly, the usefulness of his recommended communication with the family doctor would be limited in countries in which primary care medicine takes a less prominent role. Moreover, multidisciplinary documentation and assiduous record-keeping rely heavily on nursing, paraprofessional, and clerical resources that are not universally available.

In the same way, some of the investigations recommended in the English-language literature, such as analysis of body fluid samples for surreptitiously-administered medications and the use of police forensic laboratories, presuppose the existence of appropriate facilities — as do the unnecessary tests that typically precede detection of MSBP. The use of CVS to establish the diagnosis and provide evidence for court proceedings is also limited to countries in which this technology is readily available. As far as we are aware, recommendations for the use of CVS have not arisen in non-Western countries.

The details of the proposed management of mother–child separation, of the confrontation with the alleged perpetrator, and of the involvement of the non-abusing parent may be considerably affected by the roles and expectations of mothers, fathers, and extended families within different cultures. Many countries besides the United States and the United Kingdom have child abuse procedures which can be invoked to provide both separation of the child from the mother as a diagnostic tool and protection of the child once abuse is established. Countries will, however, vary in the extent to which formal legal structures have been developed, police or social services agencies become involved, and the clinician is obliged to report suspected abuse. It is clear to us that statutory structures do exist for cases of MSBP that arise in France (Bouden *et al.*, 1996; Krebs *et al.*, 1996), Italy (Caruso *et al.*, 1989; Mengarda *et al.*, 1995), Denmark (Skau and Mouridsen, 1995), Norway (Hertz *et al.*, 1995), and Germany (Marcus *et al.*, 1995a, 1995b), but we suspect that the separation of perpetrator and victim must be achieved by other means elsewhere. For example, there is no structured national system to deal with child abuse in Saudi Arabia (Al Ayed *et al.*, 1998). A reading of Meadow's (1985) recommendations makes it clear that the particular statutory measures taken in countries such as England will rely a great deal on local law. Practicing in Nigeria, however, Ifere *et al.* (1993) are explicit about the limitations of their local services, referring to "our poorly developed legal and social services with regard to the abused child"; indeed, they conclude their paper with a plea for greater resources. Among the resources that will be limited in developing countries are multidisciplinary teams of professionals, specialists such as child psychiatrists and pediatric forensic pathologists, and resources for the psychiatric treatment of perpetrators.

CONCLUSION

Despite its limitations, this review of the professional literature clearly demonstrates that MSBP is of concern internationally. A handful of English-speaking countries now accounts for the majority of the reports, but the growing number of MSBP reports from non-English-speaking and developing countries appears to be following the trend established in countries such as England and the United States: growing awareness of the phenomenon as a form of abuse is followed by increased detection, communication of findings, syntheses of case reports, and provision of recommendations based on local laws and resources. The next step — development of a community of experts who work to achieve consensus regarding matters such as optimal definition, investigation, and intervention — is one that is currently proceeding apace in the United States, United Kingdom, and elsewhere.

To date, presentations of MSBP appear largely consistent internationally. Conceptualisation of MSBP as a phenomenon of "medicalised" societies is refuted by reports from settings such as Sri Lanka and Nigeria, though cases there may increase if there is heightened Western influence. As in other forms of abuse, however, the frequency of MSBP may vary as much within as among cultures.

The literature from the United States, United Kingdom, Canada, Australia, and New Zealand often presupposes ready access to formal medical records, multidisciplinary teams, subspecialists, sophisticated diagnostic testing, and both social service agencies and legal systems dedicated to child protection. Since such resources may be seriously constrained in other countries, the contributions of professionals elsewhere will be vital in ensuring that the efforts in English-speaking industrialised settings to develop standards of care encompass an international perspective as well.

REFERENCES

Adriaenssens, P., *et al.* (1991). *Kind en Adolescent* **12**: 185–188.

Al Ayed, I. H. (1998). *Ann. Saudi Med.* **18**: 125–131.

Al-Jumaah, S., *et al.* (1993). *Ann. Saudi Med.* **13**: 469–471.

Amirali, E. L. (1998). *Can. J. Psychiatry* **43**: 632–635.

Artingstall, K. (1998). *Practical Aspects of Munchausen by Proxy and Munchausen Syndrome Investigation* (CRC Press, Boca Raton, Florida).

Barrachini, A., *et al.* (1995). *Minerva Pediatr.* **47**: 73–76.

Ben-Chetrit E., Melmed R. N. (1998). *J. Intern. Med.* 175–178.

Berthier, M., Oriot, D. (1996). *Arch. Paediatr.* **3**: 1048–1052.

Bhatia, R. S. (1990). *J. Assoc. Physicians India* **38**: 514.

Bocquet, N., *et al.* (1997). *Arch. Pediatr.* **4**: 770–778.

Bools, C. N., *et al.* (1992). *Arch. Dis. Child.* **67**: 77–79.

Bouden, A., *et al.* (1996). *Presse Med.* **25**: 567–569.

Byard, R. W., Beal, S. M. (1993). *J. Paediatr. Child Health* **29**: 77–79.

Caffey, J. (1946). *A.J.R.* **56**: 163–173.

Carlson, J., *et al.* (1994). *Acta Paediatr.* **83**: 119–121.

Caruso, M., *et al.* (1989). *Minerva Pediatr.* **41**: 525–528.

Cavenaugh, M. L. (1995). *Mommy's Little Angels* (Onyx, New York).

Chantada, G., *et al.* (1994). *Pediatr. Infect. Dis. J.* **13**: 260–263.

Clinical Psychiatry News (October 1993), 21.

D'Avanzo, M., *et al.* (1995). *Pediatr. Nephrol.* **9**: 749–750.

Davies, N. (1993). *Murder on Ward Four* (Chatto & Windus, England).

Davis, P., *et al.* (1998). *Arch. Dis. Child.* **78**: 217–221.

deRidder L., *et al.* (1988). *Ned. Tijidschr Geneeskd* **142**: 2769–2772.

DeToni, T., *et al.* (1987). *Minerva Pediatr.* **39**: 33.

Donald, T., Jureidini, J. (1996). *Arch. Pediatr. Adolesc. Med.* **150**: 753–758.

Douchain, R. (1987). *Presse Med.* **16**: 179.

Egginton, J. (1989). *From Cradle to Grave* (Morrow, New York).

Elkind, P. (1990). *The Death Shift* (Onyx, New York).

Eminson, D. M., Postlethwaite, R. J. (1992). *Arch. Dis. Child.* **67**: 1510–1516.

Eminson, D. M., Postlethwaith, R. J. (1999). *Munchausen Syndrome by Proxy: Fabricated Illness in Children* (Butterworth-Heinemann, Oxford.)

Feenstra, J., *et al.* (1988). *Tijdschrift Voor Kindergeneeskd* **56**: 148–153.

Feldman, M. D. (1994). *Int. J. Psychiatry Med.* **24**: 121–128.

Feldman, M. D., *et al.* (1997). *Gen. Hosp. Psychiatry* **19**: 24–28.

Fernandez-Jaen, A., *et al.* (1998). *Rev. Neurol.* **26**: 772–774.

Firstman, R., Talan, J. (1997). *The Death of Innocents* (Bantam, New York).

Freyberger, H. J., Freyberger, H. (1997). *Med. Klin.* **92**: 46–48.

Garbarino, J., Ebata, A. (1983). *J. Marriage Fam.* 773–783.

Ginies, J. L., *et al.* (1989). *Arch. Fr. Pediatr.* **46**: 267–269.

Ginies, J. L., *et al.* (1996). *Arch. Pediatr.* **3**: 1048–1052.

Godding, V., Kruth, M. (1991). *Arch. Dis. Child.* **66**: 956–960.

Gomez De Terreros, I., *et al.* (1996). *Child Abuse Negl.* **20**: 613–620.

Gray, J., Bentovim, A. (1996). *Child Abuse Negl.* **20**: 655–673.

Guiraldes, E., *et al.* (1995). *Rev. Med. Chile* **123**: 874–879.

Gunter, M., Boos, R. (1994). *Nervenarzt* **65**: 307–312.

Hertz, S., *et al.* (1995). *Nord. Med.* **110**: 102–104.

Hoorntje, T. M., *et al.* (1999). *Ned. Tijdschr Geneeskd* **143**: 1966–1969.

Honjo, S. (1996). *Int. J. Eating Disord.* **40**: 433–437.

Hulstijn-Dirkmaat, G. M., *et al.* (1987). *Nederlands Tiudschrift Voor Geneeskunde* **131**: 2372.

Ifere, O. A., *et al.* (1993). *Ann. Trop. Pediatr.* **13**: 281–284.

Janofsky, J. S. (1986). *J. Nerv. Ment. Dis.* **174**: 368–370.

Jimenez Hernandez, J. L., *et al.* (1987). *Actas Luso-Esp. Neurol. Psiquiatr. Cienc. Afines* **15**: 333–343.

Jimenez Hernandez, J. L., Figuerido-Poulain, J. L. (1996). *Actas Luso-Esp. Neurol. Psiquiatr. Cienc. Afines* **24**: 29–32.

Jones, D. P. (1996). *Child Abuse Negl.* **20**: 983–984.

Jureidini, J. (1993). *J. Nerv. Ment. Dis.* **181**: 135–137.

Kaufman, K. L., *et al.* (1989). *Child Abuse Negl.* **13**: 141–147.

Kaufman-Walther, V., Laederach-Hofmann, K. (1997). *Schweiz Rundsch. Mex. Prax.* **86**: 850–855.

Kennedy, R., Coombe, P. (1995). *Bull. Australian Assoc. Group Psychother.* **15**: 1–8.

Koopman, H. M., Feenstra, J. (1988). *Tijdschrift Voor Kindergeneeskd* **56**: 141–148.

Krebs, M. O., *et al.* (1996). *Presse Med.* **6**: 583–586.

Krupinski, M., *et al.* (1995). *Nervenarzt* **66**: 36–40.

Ksiazkyk, J., *et al.* (1990). *Polski Tygodnik Lekarski* **45**: 355.

Lee, A. L. (1979). *Arch. Dis. Child.* **54**: 646–647.

Lerner, V., Witztum, E., (1998). *Harefuah* **134**: 114–116.

Lesnik Oberstein, M. (1986). *Ned. Tijdschr. Geneesk.* **130**: 221–222.

Levin, A. V., Sheridan, M. S. (1995). *Munchausen Syndrome by Proxy: Issues in Diagnosis and Treatment* (Lexington, New York).

Light, M. J., Sheridan, M. S. (1990). *Clin. Pediatr.* **29**: 162–168.

Lim, L. C., *et al.* (1991). *J. Singapore Paediatr. Soc.* **33**: 59–62.

Loredo-Abdala, A., *et al.* (1991). *Bol. Med. Hosp. Infant Mex.* **48**: 121–125.

Makar, A. F., Squier, P. J. (1991). *Am. J. Pediatr.* **85**: 370–373.

Marcus, A., *et al.* (1995). *Eur. Child Adolesc. Psychiatry* **4**: 229–236.

Marcus, A., *et al.* (1995). *Child Abuse Negl.* **19**: 833–836.

Martinovic, Z. (1995). *Seizure* **4**: 129–134.

McClure, R. J., *et al.* (1996). *Arch. Dis. Child.* **75**: 57–61.

Meadow, R. (1977). *Lancet* **2**: 343–345.

Meadow, R. (1985). *Arch. Dis. Child.* **60**: 385–393.

Meadow, R. (1993). *Arch. Dis. Child.* **68**: 444–447.

Meadow, R. (1995). *Arch. Dis. Child.* **72**: 534–538.

Meadow, R. (1999). *Arch. Dis. Child.* **80**: 7–14.

Mengarda, G., *et al.* (1995). *Pediatr. Medi. Chir.* **17**: 107–110.

Mitchell, I., *et al.* (1993). *Pediatrics* **92**: 810–814.

Moszkowicz, M., Bjørnholm, K. I. (1998). *Acta Paediatr.* **87**: 601–602.

Olsen, G. (1995). *Mockingbird* (Warner Books, New York).

Ostfeld, B. M., Feldman, M. D. (1996). *Gen. Hosp. Psychiatry* **18**: 113–116.

Ostfeld, B. M., Feldman, M. D. (1996). *The Spectrum of Factitious Disorders,* eds. Feldman, M. D. and Eisendrath, S. J. (American Psychiatric Press, Washington, DC), 83–108.

Oyelami, O. A., *et al.* (1994). *Cent. Afr. Med. J.* **40**: 222–226.

Palomeque, A., *et al.* (1986). *An. Esp. Pediatr.* **25**: 256–259.

Parnell, T. F., Day, D. O. (1997). *Munchausen by Proxy Syndrome* (Sage, New York).

Perera, H., *et al.* (1995). *Ceylon Med. J.* **40**: 116–118.

Pickford, E., *et al.* (1988). *Med. J. Australia* **148**: 646–650.

Porter, G. E., *et al.* (1984). *Child Abuse Negl.* **18**: 789–794.

Prakken, A. B., *et al.* (1991). *Tijdschr Kindergeneeskd* **59**: 91–94.

Rahilly, P. M. (1991). *J. Paediatr. Child Health* **27**: 349–353.

Rand, D. C., Feldman, M. D., (1999). *Harv Rev. Psychiatry* **7**: 94–101.

Reig del Moral, *et al.* (1986). *An. Esp. Pediatr.* **25**: 251–256.

Repper, J. (1995). *J. Adv. Nurs.* **21**: 299–304.

Rogers, D., *et al.* (1976). *Br. Med. J.* **1**: 793–796.

Rosenberg, D. (1987). *Child Abuse Negl.* **11**: 547–563.

Roth, D. (1990). *Isr. J. Psychiatry Relat. Sci.* **27**: 160–167.

Samuels, M. P. (1993). *Br. Med. J.* **306**: 489–492.

Senocak, M. I., *et al.* (1995). *J. Pediatr. Surg.* **30**: 1732–1734.

Shinebourne, E. A. (1996). *J. Med. Ethics* **22**: 26–31.

Shnaps, Y., *et al.* (1981). *Pediatrics* **68**: 119–121.

Schreier, H. A., Libow, J. A. (1993). *Am. J. Orthopsychiatry* **63**: 318–321.

Schreier, H. A., Libow, J. A. (1993). *Hurting for Love* (Guilford, New York).

Sigal, M., *et al.* (1990). *Med. Law* **9**: 739–749.

Sigal, M., *et al.* (1989). *Comp. Psychiatry* **30**: 527–533.

Sigal, M., *et al.* (1991). *Isr. J. Psychiatry Relat. Sci.* **28**: 33–36.

Sigal, M. D., *et al.* (1986). *J. Nerv. Ment. Dis.* **174**: 696–698.

Skau, K., Mouridsen, S. E. (1995). *Acta Paediatr.* **84**: 977–982.

Smith, N. J., Ardern, M. H. (1989). *J. Fam. Ther.* **11**: 321–334.

Solami, V. K., (1998). *Int. J. Dermatol.* **37**: 229–230.

Sugar, J. A., *et al.* (1991). *J. Am. Acad. Child Adolesc. Psychiatry* **30**: 1015–1021.

The Atlanta Journal and Constitution, 21 July 1995, D1.

The Guardian, 18 May 1993, 2.

The Lancet **4** (1994), 1373–1374.

Thomas, T. J. (1996). *Med. Ethics* **22**: 22–25.

Vondrak, K., *et al.* (1995). *Cas. Lek. Cesk.* **134**: 349–350.

Vouzemoix (1995). *Rev. Med. Suisse Romande* **115**: 513–514.

Warner, J. O., Hathaway, M. J. (1983). *Arch. Dis. Child.* **59**: 463–464.

Wright, N. (1984). *A Mother's Trial* (Bantam, New York).

Yorker, B. C. (1995). *Health Matrix* **5**: 325–346.

Yorker, B. C. (1996). *The Spectrum of Factitious Disorders*, eds. Feldman, M. D. and Eisendrath, S. J. (American Psychiatric Press, Washington, DC), 157–174.

Zahner, J., Schneider, W. (1994). *Dtsch. Med. Wochenschr.* **119**: 192–195.

CHAPTER 3

Child Abuse Specific to the Medical System

JON JUREIDINI
Head, Department of Psychological Medicine,
Women's & Children's Hospital, Adelaide

TERRY DONALD
Head, Child Protection Service,
Women's & Children's Hospital, Adelaide

The term Munchausen Syndrome by Proxy was first used to identify a particular form of behaviour by a parent that led to the creation in their child of symptoms and/or signs that were indistinguishable from those that would have been seen if the child had suffered from non-induced disease. Because that behaviour was harmful to the child, it was correctly considered to be a serious form of child abuse. In the original cases that were called Munchausen Syndrome by Proxy, the behaviour of the parent (mother) towards her child was strongly and directly influenced by the responses of the doctor (most often a subspecialist paediatrician) to the child's apparently undiagnosable disease, so that symptom induction by the mother seemed to be timed to maintain the doctor's interest in and fascination with the "case". By common paediatric usage, the term Munchausen Syndrome by Proxy (MSBP) is now often used, not only to refer to the classical cases described above, but also to any situation in which a parent in some way appears to compromise the medical care of her child. Examples include parental overtreating or undertreating of such medical conditions as asthma, epilepsy and cystic fibrosis. In these latter examples the relationship with the doctor is different from that described above, often being characterised more by a dependency on the doctor by the parent who manifests an unusually high level of anxiety towards her child's illness, which may be relatively mild to moderate in its true severity. Our usage of the term will be consistent with the original. In this chapter, we will set some of the ambiguities about diagnosis into historical perspective, identify some ongoing areas of uncertainty, and discuss the special role of the medical system in this form of child abuse.

First, we address the differentiation of the behaviour that rightly is designated MSBP from other forms of child abuse, and the implications for diagnostic practice. MSBP differs from some other forms of abuse in that it is premeditated rather than impulsive, and is not apparently reactive to the child's behaviour, but neither of these features is unique to MSBP (characterising, e.g., much child sexual abuse). Similarly, the perpetrator's behaviour at presentation does not neatly distinguish MSBP from other forms of abuse. For instance, most children who are physically abused by their parent(s) are presented for medical attention, the perpetrator rarely admitting his/her role in causing the injuries. The diagnosis of physical abuse is not based on the "profile" of the suspected abusers but on the nature of the injury, the age of the child and the plausability of apparent mechanisms of injury inferred from the explanation provided by the parents. Similarly for MSBP, when a child's symptoms or signs are not attributable to any "natural disease", they may be considered to have been fabricated and attributable to parental behaviour. However, MSBP behaviour can produce symptoms/signs which are indistinguishable from those resulting from the occurrence of a natural disease, so that there is a greater chance with this form of abuse that doctors will continue to try and identify an elusive natural disease process. This search subjects the child to expensive and sometimes dangerously invasive investigations. In the seminal cases of MSBP, doctors vigorously pursued new diseases to explain the symptoms, not realising that they were part of an interaction with an abusive parent who was continually reinforcing the lack of a definitive diagnosis by persistently re-creating symptoms in the child. As a reaction to the increasingly broad and somewhat haphazard use of the label "Munchausen by Proxy", there have been arguments for dispensing with the term, and classifying cases of children presenting with apparently spurious symptoms according to the nature of the symptoms and a statement relating to their apparent cause (Morley, 1995; Fisher, 1995). Thus, just as the most appropriate way to describe a case of physical abuse is to describe the injury or damage from the perspective of the victim (e.g., fractured femur, secondary to assault), then so might we refer to the abusive induction of symptoms/signs by specifically describing the symptoms. This approach is followed to some extent by Samuels *et al.* (1992) in their use of the term "Imposed Upper Airway Obstruction", whilst Bools (1996) goes further and suggests that not only the abusive behaviour should be described but also the act of fabrication and any psychiatric diagnosis in the perpetrator.

Another important historical thread to be aware of in understanding current difficulties with MSBP is the inconsistency from its first usage as to whether the term applies to the parent (Meadow, 1977), the child (Money and Werlwas, 1976) or both. Current practice is usually to attach the label to the perpetrator, but ambiguity continues. It is plausible that there is something characteristic about the perpetrator of MSBP, perhaps even some common pattern of psychiatric disturbance, but MSBP behaviour itself is clearly not an intrinsic characteristic of an individual. The attribution of the label of MSBP to a parent implies that there has been an active interaction between the parent (perpetrator) and medical professionals which has contributed to the child's clinical condition and therefore the manifestations of the abusive behaviour. However, the use of the label MSBP to describe behaviour does not and should not be taken to imply something inherent in the individual responsible for the behaviour. This point has important implications in the management of children who are abused in this way, particularly in regard to their future safety. For instance, Meadow (1985) has made the point that psychiatrists who carry out assessments on parents who are believed to have demonstrated MSBP behaviour may pronounce the parent to be healthy, and therefore free of the illness of MSBP. Such a conclusion carries the implication that the mother could not have carried out the abuse and therefore that abuse has not occurred.

Concerns about to whom the label applies, along with the failure to clearly identify MSBP as child abuse led a task force of the American

Professional Society on the Abuse of Children to attempt, in 1995, to "clarify the constellation of behaviours described as Munchausen by Proxy (MBP)". The task force attempted to clarify the MBP position by separating out Paediatric Condition Falsification (PCF) and Factitious Disorder by Proxy (FDP). They defined PCF as a form of child maltreatment in which an adult falsifies physical and/or psychological signs and/or symptoms in a child victim. FDP, on the other hand was to be a psychiatric diagnosis applied to adult perpetrators who intentionally falsify history, signs or symptoms in a victim (usually a child) to meet their own self-serving psychological needs. The task force included under the heading "abuse by PCF" such situations as children who are abused by their parents who then lie about the circumstances of the child's illness; children who are neglected or fail to thrive due to the inability of the parent to cope with the child; "help seeking" parents who are overwhelmed and falsify symptoms to get assistance in caring for their child, none of which would then be classified as examples of Factitious Disorder by Proxy. In our view, this definition of PCF is too broad, encompassing much of child abuse. Furthermore, it is important to remember that parents can have abnormal reactions to illness in their children without that constituting child abuse. Finally, the task force gives insufficient weight to the necessity of active involvement of a paediatric specialist in the diagnostic interaction with the parent in cases of FDP.

Indeed, none of the most widely accepted definitions of Munchausen Syndrome by Proxy sufficiently emphasise the centrality of the relationship between the abusive behaviour and the medical system, and we will therefore now examine the implications of our view that behaviour that can legitimately be called MSBP is carried out by a parent but is necessarily in concert with the medical system. The special relationship between perpetrator and medical system is maintained and developed by the abusive parent continuing to deny responsibility for the production of symptoms or disease, the motivation being apparently something other than the desire to avoid the consequences of their abusive behaviour. For example, as we have previously pointed out, the condition referred to as Imposed Upper Airway Obstruction (IUAO) should not be considered a manifestation of MSBP behaviour unless the perpetrator seeks a relationship with the medical system (Donald and

Jureidini, 1996). Often the child who suffers IUAO is only presented to hospital for acute treatment, the engagement with the medical system in such cases being identical to that seen when any child is presented with a serious illness or injury, or life threatening event. It is important to note, however, that MSBP behaviour may not always begin as an attempt to engage the medical system. In some cases, the gratification which may be gained from having an ill child is learned by a parent as they interact with the system of modern medicine, for example, when their child has a genuine illness; or when through the effects of their previous abusive behaviour they succeed in misleading doctors into accepting that their child's condition has resulted from an accident or the effects of a true disease.

Another significant problem with existing diagnostic criteria for MSBP is the difficulty caused by having to make judgements about motivation. For example, the American Psychiatric Association's Diagnostic and Statistical Manual (1994) includes amongst its criteria for "Factitious Disorder by Proxy" that "the motivation for the perpetrator's behaviour is to assume the sick role by proxy". Whilst it might be reasonable to infer, on the basis of clinical observations, that a perpetrator actively seeks some involvement with the medical system, in the vast majority of cases, it is not possible to clearly understand the perpetrator's motivation in doing so. We have therefore proposed modifications to the diagnostic criteria for MSBP to explicitly specify the characteristic three-way transaction that actively involves the doctor, parent (as perpetrator) and child (as victim), as well as the factitious nature of the denial of the abusive behaviour by the perpetrator. Diagnosis requires:

1. Fabrication or induction of illness in order to facilitate involvement with the medical system, by a care-giver(s), who then
2. Denies responsibility for that illness, which is
3. Misattributed by doctors to some medical cause(s), not necessarily clearly defined.

The last criterion emphasises the importance of medical misdiagnosis, and implies that the factitious illness is ultimately resolved by it being correctly recognised as fabricated. More commonly however, doctors continue to be misled by the perpetrator, often with escalation in illness, as diagnostic uncertainty leads to further investigations and often multiple hit or miss treatment interventions.

However, adopting our more stringent definition does not obviate all of the definitional ambiguities around MSBP. The question arises as to how direct the perpetrator's interaction with the medical system needs to be. For example, a recently published article was co-written by a woman who had been, between the ages of two and ten, the victim of severe physical abuse by her mother (Bryk and Siegel, 1997). The abusing mother had inflicted broken bones and infection on her daughter by a regime of non-impulsive, apparently pre-meditated assaults, including hammer blows, the introduction of foreign substances into the child's body and the scalding of the child with boiling water. There was enough evidence of engagement with the medical system to justify the label "MSBP", and without the daughter's first hand account, it may have seemed that all of her behaviour was directed to that end. However, the victim's reports demonstrates that a good deal of the abusive behaviour took place outside of the hospital setting. The victim reported her earliest memory as being tied into a high chair whilst her mother hit her on the foot with a hammer, and she recalled her mother justifying the behaviour by saying "I am doing this for your own good. The doctor wants me to do this treatment to make you better." From the victim's perspective as an adult, her mother's love for her "was connected to hurting me and keeping me sick", and it is by no means clear that her mother's behaviour was primarily driven by her interaction with the medical system. We therefore question how much abuse might occur in other cases of MSBP that is not directly driven by the desire for medical engagement. A second question is whether the label MSBP should be used in situations of illness/symptom induction in which it becomes apparent that the motivation is at least partly understandable in other ways. In the above case, that additional motivation might have been sadism whilst in other cases, partial explanation might come from financial rewards from illness, or where relationship problems between parents lead to an indirect attack on the partner through abusive behaviour towards the child (Rogers *et al.*, 1976).

With these unanswered questions, the final point to be considered is the special role that the medical system plays in the genesis and maintenance of MSBP. There is a considerable literature on the special relationship between MSBP perpetrators and their doctors and a number of authors have drawn attention to the role of doctors and nurses in the exacerbation and perpetuation of MSBP (Morley, 1995; Fisher and Mitchell, 1995; Zitelli *et al.*, 1987; Sigal *et al.*, 1989; Schreier, 1992; Meadow, 1995). We contend that doctors and nurses are *central* to the aetiology of MSBP. The MSBP scenario arises where relatively unsophisticated history-taking leads to misjudgements about the most likely explanation for symptoms, and thoughtful consideration is to some extent replaced by investigative and diagnostic zeal, perhaps a product of the increasing objectification of the body (Redding, 1995). The abusive behaviour identified as MSBP can therefore be seen as highlighting some of the failings of modern technological medicine, because in addition to requiring a parent who has both the capacity for abuse (Finkelhor, 1984) and the potential to be gratified by the medical system, MSBP depends for its existence on a medical system which is highly sub-specialised, investigation oriented and fascinated by rare conditions. The apparently recent evolution of MSBP can not only be seen as resulting from technological, but also from sociological and litigious changes in medical practice in our society (Meadow, 1994). Freer visiting arrangements and increased consultation with parents are clearly positive advances in paediatric medical practice, but they have also played a role in the facilitation of parents' ability to carry out this form of abuse in hospital. Parents often advocate for additional treatments and investigations, and paediatricians are vulnerable to pressures from them to provide answers. The medical fear of missing serious, diagnosable illness means that parents can be very influential in directing medical investigation, especially when the continuing search for a disease diagnosis obscures the abusive parental behaviour. Doctors work on the assumption that the patient/parent tells the truth because they wish to optimise the chance of their child's recovery. In a "natural disease process" this assumption assists the diagnostic process, but in the face of induced or fabricated symptoms, it minimises the chance that the true nature of the medical condition will be realised and drives the doctor to investigate further.

Cases have been seen in which the doctor and the parent have seemed equally excited by the unusual and apparently rare nature of illness, and individual doctors have been known to be the treating physician in more than one case of MSBP. These observations leads us to close with a final speculation — that there may be specific characteristics of doctors that predispose them to becoming engaged in a case of MSBP. The potential "MSBP doctor" might be a competent and well respected paediatrician, but one who tends to see things in black and white terms, for example, wanting to understand problems as either all medical or all psychosocial. He/she would be likely to work in an area of paediatrics where diagnostic certainty is rare and be dependent upon multiple medical investigations. A high level of investigatory zeal might come, in part, from anxiety about missing the diagnosis, but also from an attraction to the possibility of establishing a rare diagnosis that colleagues have missed. Such doctors may be more vulnerable than their peers to becoming caught up in the MSBP scenario. We would emphasise the importance of considering this explanation early, and consulting widely, as precautionary measures.

REFERENCES

American Psychiatric Association (1994). *Diagnostic and Statistical Manual of Mental Disorders (4th Edition): DSM IV.* American Psychiatric Association.

Bools, C. (1996). Factitious Illness by Proxy: Munchausen Syndrome by Proxy. *Br. J. Psych.* **169**: 268–275.

Bryk, M., Siegel, P. (1997). My mother caused my illness: The story of a survivor of Munchausen by Proxy Syndrome. *Pediatrics* **100**: 1–7.

Definitional Issues in Munchausen by Proxy. APSAC Task Force Report. The APSAC Advisor **11** (1998) 7–10.

Donald, T., Jureidini, J. (1996). Munchausen by Proxy Syndrome: Child abuse in the medical system. *Arch. Pediatr. Adolesc. Health* **150**: 753–758.

Finkelhor, D. (1984). *Child Sexual Abuse.* (The Free Press, New York).

Fisher, G., Mitchell, I. (1995). Is Munchausen Syndrome by Proxy really a syndrome? *Arch. Dis. Child.* **72**: 530–534.

Meadow, R. (1977). Munchausen Syndrome by Proxy: The hinterland of child abuse. *Lancet* **2(8033)**: 343–345.

Meadow, R. (1985). Management of Munchausen Syndrome by Proxy. *Arch. Dis. Child.* **60**: 385–393.

Meadow, S. R. (1994). Who's to blame — mothers, Munchausen or medicine? *J. R. Coll. Physicians Lond.* **28**: 332–337.

Meadow, R. (1995). What is, and what is not, "Munchausen Syndrome by Proxy"? *Arch. Dis. Child.* **72**: 534–538.

Money, J., Werlwas, J. (1976). *Folie a deux* in the parents of psychosocial dwarfs: Two cases. *Bull. Am. Acad. Psychiatry Law* **4**: 51–62.

Morley, C. (1995). Practical concerns about the diagnosis of Munchausen Syndrome by Proxy. *Arch. Dis. Child.* **72**: 528–529.

Redding, P. (1995). Science, medicine, and illness: Rediscovering the patient as a person. In *Troubled Bodies: Critical Perspectives on Postmodernism, Medical Ethics, and the Body*, ed. Komesaroff, P. (Duke University Press, Durham).

Rogers, D., Tripp, J., Bentovim, A., Robinson, A., Berry, D., Goulding, R. (1976). Non-accidental poisoning: An extended form of child abuse. *Br. Med. J.* **1**: 793–796.

Samuels, M., McClaughlin, W., Jacobson, R., Poets, C., Southall, D. (1992). Fourteen cases of imposed upper airways obstruction. *Arch. Dis. Child.* **67**: 162–170.

Schreier, H. (1992). The perversion of mothering: Munchausen Syndrome by Proxy. *Bull. Menninger Clin.* **56**: 421–437.

Sigal, M., Gelkopf, M., Meadow, R. (1989). Munchausen by Proxy Syndrome: The triad of abuse, self-abuse, and deception. *Comp. Psychiatry* **30**: 527–533.

Zitelli, B., Seltman, M., Shannon, R. (1987). Munchausen's Syndrome by Proxy and its professional participants. *Am. J. Dis. Child.* **141**: 1099–1102.

CHAPTER 4

The Extraordinary Case of Mrs H.

ESTELA V. WELLDON
Consultant Psychiatrist,
Portman Clinic and Honorary Senior Lecturer in Forensic Psychotherapy,
University of London

Notwithstanding my large clinical experience of dealing with mothers who exhibit the most damaging and perverse attitudes towards their children (Welldon, 1988), I found myself in a state of disbelief and shock when I was asked to prepare a psychiatric court report on Mrs H. Such was the horror of Mrs H's actions that left me astounded, confused and unable to think. Mrs H was suspected of pulling and removing, from birth, her two babies' finger and toenails. At the time of the enquiry they were aged 21 months and ten months. A case of Munchausen Syndrome by Proxy was suspected and an assessment of her parenting abilities, with the confirmation of this diagnosis and her suitability for psychotherapy, was needed.

During psychiatric assessments, mothers usually display strong emotions about the possibility of their children being taken away and try very hard to give a "good impression" of their maternal abilities. This was not the case with Mrs H. who appeared all throughout our meetings to be completely devoid of any feelings; flat in her affects, detached and disassociated. Not even when she said: "the most important thing in my life are my children and I want them back with me" did she show any signs of affection.

Another unusual feature in this case was that the removal of her children's toe and fingernails, appeared to be a cold planned revenge, showing a strong sadistic quality. In contrast, previous cases involved mothers who had become impulsive, out of control and aggressive during the course of their mothering duties. There were no precedents of this kind of behaviour except in acts of torture.

MRS H'S STORY

Whereas at the beginning Mrs H. denied harming her children, she eventually told me that not only had she done so, but that also, whilst harming them, she was effectively able to convince all professionals involved, general practitioners and paediatricians, that the children's suffering was the result of skin diseases. I consider that, in some ways, she must have felt seriously distressed about being able to deceive all the professionals, because she knew that those actions were extremely harmful to her children and to herself; because she was getting away with it when she was in urgent need of professional help.

These actions could easily and vividly evoke the Medea complex; but cannot be solely and simply explained as a vengeful strategy against an "uncaring" husband. I hypothesise that her strong sense of revenge was born in early infancy and directed, symbolically speaking, first against her own mother for abandoning her at four months, and later against her father for sexually abusing her from the age of six. These explosive negative feelings had been enacted in a combination of neglect and abuse towards her own children from their birth culminating in the most unthinkable sadistic behaviour.

Compulsions to enact, as opposed to experience, feelings are linked to early traumas where mother–baby bonding breaks down at early stages of the baby's emotional development. Being the receptacle of early neglect and abuse had seriously impeded Mrs H's mothering function. It seemed as if being confronted with evidence that she could produce healthy babies, produced a type of disbelief in her about herself. She could not accept any intrinsic goodness in herself because this would implicitly imply a recognition that she was intact, despite the injurious harm inflicted by her own mother, and a denial of damage. This lead her, in turn, to inflict on her healthy babies endless suffering and serious bodily damage.

When I began to regain my capacity for thought, I speculated that taking away growing and protective structures, (such as nails) leaving fragile, raw skin exposed to continuous physical harm, might indicate the way she experienced herself; as a raw object, exposed to so much suffering that she had to rigidly protect herself with detachment and strangeness to avoid experiencing her own unbearable pain.

MOTHERHOOD, ABUSE AND PERVERSION

Elsewhere, (Welldon, 1988; Welldon, 1999) I have described female perversions as either self-abuse or child abuse, which then becomes a dual process involving mother and baby. In general, female perversion is very different from male perversion because women direct their aim towards themselves, their bodies or what they perversely regard as an extension of themselves, their babies. In contrast, mens' unconscious sadism is directed towards an outside object or target. The object in women is highly cathexed physical and emotional attachments. This characteristic, again, is in contrast to men who do not experience the same emotional or physical investment. Female perversions include bulimia, anorexia, self-mutilation, sexual and physical abuse of children, including incest with their children of both sexes.

It seems to have been difficult to accept the notion of perverse motherhood and other female perverse behaviour; despite the completely different psychopathology which originates from the female body and its inherent attributes. However, motherhood provides an excellent vehicle for some women to exercise perverse and perverting attitudes towards their offspring in unconscious retaliation against their own mothers. Some of the most common findings among perverse women include an early history of abandonment and neglect, and experience of either physical or sexual abuse or both.

Some women who feel inadequate and insecure experience their child as the only available source of emotional nourishment, and demand that they satisfy their craving for physical affection. It is well known that incestuous mothers do not facilitate, indeed, do not allow from their infants any process of individuation and or separation. Actually, the opposite holds true, they use that baby as a part of themselves, almost in a fetish-like fashion. Most of our patients who suffer from perversions have a history of an engulfing relationship with their mothers with repeated switches to neglect and abandonment.

Prior to presenting the problem of being perpetrators of child abuse, most women have a history of self-abuse. This is often manifest during adolescence in the form of eating disorders, such as anorexia and bulimia, promiscuity, drug abuse, self cutting and burning. A pregnancy at an early age, coinciding with their own mothers' age at pregnancy is not unusual. Pregnancies as an outcome of a sense of inadequacy, hatred or revenge, (conscious or unconscious), or a "quick replacement pregnancy" can also lead to child abuse. Lack of emotional and practical resources during pregnancy and early mothering is often the case, as well as associations with uncaring and violent men leading to sado-masochistic relationships. These could also involve other women.

In women the onset of perversion is usually stress related. They have much more flexibility than their male counterparts in displaying their perverse symptomatology. It is not uncommon for women to go through different stages of self-abuse and abuse to children; their own or others, in a different fashion to their male counterparts: this can be seen in male paedophilia in which men experience a complete lack of inner freedom in the "choice" of their psychopathology. In women, perverse psychopathology can disappear completely for long periods of time and then abruptly starts again, usually under new situations of pressure or stress.

Perversion of motherhood is the end product of serial abuse or chronic infantile neglect. This condition involves at least three generations in which faulty and inadequate mothering perpetuates itself in a circular motion reproducing a cycle of abuse. It occurs as a breakdown of inner mental structures: the mother feels not only emotionally crippled in dealing with all those huge psychological and physical demands from her baby, but also impotent and unable to obtain gratification from other sources. She perceives the world around her as non-existent in any helpful or supporting way. It is then that she falls back on inappropriate and perverse behaviour: this, in turn, makes her feel powerless and unable to cope with her unhappy baby. Simultaneously and paradoxically, she experiences her perverse behaviour as a mother as the only power available to her, through her exclusive emotional and physical authority over her baby.

Massive denial that women could be capable of child abuse was the rule until the 1960s when the role of mothers in "battered baby syndrome" was first recognised. Interestingly, recognition of the dangers of physical abuse of children by mothers did not come from professionals dealing with women with psychological problems, but from experienced paediatricians who could no longer ignore the suffering of the babies they were treating. A comparable situation arises with Munchausen Syndrome By Proxy; a "discovery" made by a paediatrician (Meadow, 1977).

It is the equation of motherhood and health which may lead to perpetuation of stereotypes which identify women only as victims. This in fact inhibits women from disclosing dreams of revenge, or abuse of power and the extreme need to be in control. Social powers are unequally distributed between women and men, with women's exclusive power confined to the domestic sphere where abuse is hidden away and possibilities for practical, emotional resources are not available. Men's access to public power, results in their transgressions being more public; with the "natural" concomitant of humiliation and punishment being the available resources.

The outcome of this division affects individuals and society in general. Women are to be the only victims, and treated with sedatives, and men are always the perpetrators, faced with "penalisation" and punishment. Thus perverse behaviour is very much intertwined with the politics of power. Women have access to domestic power where men have access to public power.

MUNCHAUSEN SYNDROME BY PROXY AS PERVERSION IN WOMEN

Initially, I questioned the inclusion of Munchausen Syndrome by Proxy in my definition of female perversion, because at first sight, it appeared to involve three persons: a mother, a child and a medical practitioner. Within this triangular relationship, the medical practitioner's clinical judgement is corrupted or perverted by the mother's ability to persuade him (and it usually is a he) that her baby's physical ill health is caused by fictitious illnesses.

In Mother, Madonna, Whore I identified the process of MBPS as a symbolically dual one between the doctor and the mother, since the mother is in complete identification with the image of a seriously ill baby. Understood in this way, the process could be defined as a form of female perversion. Despite protestations about the adequacy of this term, "by proxy" is wittingly or unwittingly the most accurate way to designate this extremely severe psychopathological syndrome; because the child is proxy for the mother's internal distress. Over the ten years since publication of Mother, Modonna, Whore, awareness of MBPS has risen and my own clinical observations identify distinctive features which differentiate MBPS and perverse mothering (1999). There are some common traits in the mothers' histories, but the differences in the mothers' attitudes and actions are important. The perverse mother may neglect or physically or sexually abuse her child. She is concerned and experiences anxiety, but is secretive about her actions and scared of being caught. Cases of MSBP always require a third party (a professional), are always premeditated, cold-blooded, show complete detachment and are always presented as seeking help. The mother will also commit at least one of four actions: smothering, poisoning, fabrication of seizures or other symptoms. Perverse mothers are often young mother, with a history of eating disorders and/or self harm. In contrast MSBP mothers tend to be older and present with somatising behaviors and/or a history of illness. The ways in which the babies are treated also differ: perverse mothers usually concern older babies who may present in future with serious personality disorders. In cases of MSBP the babies are usually much younger and they in future may have physical illness sometimes leading to death. The professional attitudes are also different: in maternal perversion the patient is usually completely isolated, her problems are met with disbelief and lack of awareness. The patient is usually amenable to treatment if offered: the assessment of parenting abilities is relatively easy in long-term assessments. Cases of MSBP usually involve many medical staff and hospitals with the focus placed on the baby's physical illness. The mother usually resists treatment and assessment of parenting abilities is difficult.

In my own theories the main difference between a male and female perverse action lies in the aim. Whereas in men the act is aimed at an outside target, in women it is usually against themselves, either against their bodies or against their babies. The inclusion in the MBPS by Shreier and Libow of a third figure, that of "an all-powerful male figure" represented by the paediatrician, provides a process of triangulation, returning in this way to the traditional phallocentric Freudian theories. This denies or ignores the importance of the relationship between mother and baby, which I believe it is the central focus of the perversion of mothering.

The case of Beverley Allitt is intriguing, since she could be considered to be in between the two different diagnostic classifications, although she is not the mother who either brings the sick child to the paediatrician nor the perverse mother who abuses her children.

As the following media descriptions show, she has the background of a perverse mother, and therefore this leads towards the diagnosis of a perversion of motherhood. "A 24 year-old nurse admits to having killed four children and attacked nine other children, all of them in her ward, under her care." At her trial, the newspapers noted that: "she was suffering from anorexia nervosa…. She had been inflicting serious injury on her own body while as a student nurse." She was also described by a Home Office forensic psychiatrist as "this very damaged lady."

There are many reasons why the Beverley Allitt case was so shocking. First, being a woman, she did not fit with the model established for other serial killers. Another factor may have been that her violence to children took place during the course of her work when she was surrounded by caring professionals, including most experienced and expert medical practitioners. Why were they so unaware of what was happening to the children involved, and the "damage" in their colleague?

The actual dangerousness in Beverley Allit case is devastatingly obvious. What are the determinants for these horrific killings? What has been overlooked and even neglected? Could this violent behaviour have been predicted earlier on? Were there circumstances which could have established a higher degree of risk which would increase the chances for this dangerousness? And further more, is this dangerousness intrinsically female? And if so, why? How can we use this awful experience to discover possible ways to improve our means of accurately detecting and assessing "dangerousness" and hence, hopefully pre-empt further criminal behaviour in the future.

FEMALE PERVERSION AND INDICATORS OF RISK

Failure to understand the nature of female perversion has led some very "damaged ladies" being so misunderstood as to be either encouraged to work with children, when they are at risk of abusing them; or denied the treatment they need and for which they sometimes plead.

It is worth noting that, many young and psychologically damaged women constantly seek working positions in the caring professions with direct access to children. There are unconscious motivations involved in the choice by young women to take on a child-caring role. At times, they are obliviously unaware of the dangers they are exposing themselves and to children which could easily produce serious consequences to all involved. As a society, we should be more attentive to monitoring process during selection procedures and be more caring and responsible in providing consistent supervision to untrained and poorly paid personnel whose difficult task is to take care of children and disabled people.

Conventional attitudes, and ignorance of female perversion, are among the reasons why it is taking so long for the profession, let alone the public, to accept that women as mothers or in mothering professions can inflict irreparable and permanent damage to the children they are supposed to care for. My clinical observations confirm this bias. On countless occasions, agencies and establishments have expressed alarm, sometimes verging on panic, when referring male patients to me as sexual abusers. This contrasts strongly with the difficulty my female patients have often had in being taken seriously by some agencies. After the publication of my book, many women referred themselves to the Portman Clinic for treatment, and told me that all their previous attempts to get professional attention for their mixed or negative feelings, and abusive activities (either emotion or physical), to their child, whether boy or girl, were not really taken seriously. So, the acknowledgement of female perversion was absent, though the evidence was that male perversion is often the result of an early faulty mothering.

After years of clinical experience, I have had to acknowledge that there are feelings and activities amongst women that could or must be called perverse, even if the mental mechanisms are different from those found in men. I am arguing that in both sexes the reproductive functions and the organs attached to them are those used for perversion; the man has the penis to carry out his perverse activities, while the woman has the whole body to pursue them, since the female reproductive-sexual organs are more widely spread.

The important differences between males and females, could help us in the prediction, assessment and management of female dangerousness. These could be used in a positive way to promote further understanding and prevention of these particular conditions. For example, in perverse women, a history of abuse to their own bodies is consistently found and outstanding. At times, the sadistic self-attack is inflicted as a means to protect the children from their own experienced dangerousness. In view of the earlier clinical findings including self-harm one could, in this particular predicament, actually suspect future female dangerousness to others. This is not to say or even to predict that self-abuse will be superseded by child abuse. However, the knowledge that these two conditions could be associated it might facilitate a better anamnesis with proper care of all involved.

In the diagnostic approach we should be aware of some crucial factors which may be linked to the present psychopathology, for example, was the particular abused child singled out from birth? Did the gender of the child created a disappointment at birth? Did she represent or re-enact another child, such as the product of a quick replacement pregnancy following the death or miscarriage of a previous child/pregnancy? Or a brother/sister that the patient felt resembled herself as a child? Did she consider abusing that child for a long time prior to the actual abuse? Or was it sudden and unexpected? Was the abuse taking place when the woman was feeling unable to convey to anyone her own sense of despair and desperation, or when she was in distress or feeling extremely isolated, helpless or moody? Did the acting out bring a temporary sense of relief and elation? Was this a chronic condition or was it aggravated by superimposed conditions? Another important characteristic to be elicited is the degree of emotional attachment that mothers feel towards the children involved in the abuse. The question should also be asked whether they are able to stop themselves from acting out these sadistic fantasies and if so, how.

CONCLUSION

It seems important to develop a personality profile which could lead to the prevention, accurate diagnosis and better treatment of these conditions. Evaluations should include number and gender in the family tree; value of femininity in the family, noting educational achievements in both girls and boys. Recording of mother's and grandmother's previous pregnancies and family known incestuous activities with short and long term consequences are important. Beverly Allit described a horrific history of self-mutilation while being a student nurse, and she was suffering from anorexia at the time of her trial. Had this new concept of female perversion been taken into account, a job involving "mothering" duties would have been clearly counter-indicated.

The inability to obtain professional help may be due to:

a) patients' enormous difficulties due to shame or
b) professionals' difficulties to listen

The reluctance to listen may be due to both a marked response of disbelief, and helplessness; or a tendency in the profession to call "problem" women, hysterics, manipulators, inadequate, attention-seekers. This response is further reinforced by society's value of glorified motherhood and the all-too-frequent equation of motherhood with good mental health. New awareness and deeper insights to women's psychopathologies are available and should be used in a positive way to promote further understanding and prevention of these particular conditions.

Management suggestions include gaining a full understanding of the woman's internal world in reference to her own gender according to previous generations and her own insights about herself as a woman and as a prospective mother. We should be alerted to women with a history of self-abuse who are seeking training positions or jobs which involve the caring professions.

A close co-operation between all those professionals who care for either mothers and/or babies is needed to secure both accurate diagnosis and adequate provisions for both MBPS and perverse mothering. This should be aimed to prevent further abuses of domestic power which cause much pain, suffering and distress to both mothers and babies in the short run and society in general in longer terms.

There is still much to be explored and researched before we can establish with any clinical confidence the state of these conditions. The three-generational approach to assessing the history of the presenting patient would appear very important in establishing some neutrality.

REFERENCES

Meadow, R. (1977). MSBP, the hinterland of child abuse. *Lancet* **2**: 343–345.

Welldon, E. (1992). *Mother, Madonna, Whore: The idealisation and denegration of motherhood.* Free Association Books, London 1988; current American Edition, Guilford Press, New York.

Welldon, E. (1992). Perversion of motherhood. In *Mother, Madona, Whore: The idealisation and denegration of motherhood.* Guilford Press, New York.

Welldon, E. (1995). Female perversion and hysteria. *Br. J. Psych.* **11(3)**: 406–414.

Welldon, E. (1996). Contrasts in male and female perversions. In *Forensic Psychotherapy*, eds. Cordess, C. and Cox, M. Jessica Kingsley Publishers, London. pp. 273–289.

Welldon, E. (2000). Review of disordered mother or disordered diagnosis? MSBP, In *Psychoanalytic Studies*, Vol. 2, No. 2, eds. Allison, D. B. and Roberts, M. S. Carfax Publishing, Taylor & Francis Ltd. pp. 193–194.

.

CHAPTER 5

Munchausen's Syndrome by Proxy: A Perspective from Primary Care

MICHAEL J. BANNON
Consultant Paediatrician,
Northwick Park & St. Marks NHS Trust, London

YVONNE H. CARTER
Professor of General Practice & Primary Care,
Queen Mary and Westfield College, London

Jamie, a six-year-old boy, presented to the accident and emergency department of a large district general hospital on several occasions with a history given by his mother that he had had a fit at home. Following referral to a paediatrician, all investigations were found to be normal. Jamie was admitted on three further occasions following further descriptions of seizures at home. His paediatrician prescribed an anti-convulsant on the basis that epilepsy may occur in children even when investigations are normal. Over the next year, Jamie was admitted on six further occasions as a result of fits. His paediatrician increased the dose of the drug and added another in order to achieve better control of the epilepsy; following this, Jamie was again admitted. On this occasion, he showed signs of drug toxicity. The case notes were reviewed by a colleague who discovered that none of the fits have been witnessed by a professional and that, on inquiry, none have been noted at Jamie's school. Following discussion with social services, a planning meeting was held at the hospital. Jamie's GP was invited but did not attend. No firm conclusions were reached at the meeting and the paediatrician was urged to discuss the case with the GP.

Following a telephone conversation between the two doctors, a further confidential planning meeting was held at the GP's surgery. The GP revealed that Jamie's mother has had treatment for a personality disorder and that Jamie has been treated for peanut allergy by the doctors at the surgery (the paediatrician was unaware of this). Social services on further investigation of the family were informed by their colleagues in another district that Jamie's older sibling was on the child protection register because of neglect and emotional abuse and that another child died at the age of four months because of "cot death". At the instigation of the paediatrician, Jamie was admitted to a specialist epilepsy unit for one month where no seizures were observed and no food allergy documented. A child protection case conference was held and Jamie's name was placed on the register because of likely significant harm (Munchausen's Syndrome by Proxy). The GP sends a written report but does not attend the conference. She later agrees to refer Jamie's mother for psychotherapy. Jamie and his brother are taken into care.

This case raises several important points for discussion. Munchausen's Syndrome by Proxy (MSBP) may be considered in terms of a triangular relationship between the child, carer (usually mother) and the doctor (Murray, 1997), (Fig. 1). The doctor's role in this context has attracted much comment in the literature on two accounts: firstly in terms of the difficulties associated with making a confident diagnosis and, secondly, with respect to unintentional complicity in the overall MSBP process as a result of inappropriate investigation of spurious symptoms and unnecessary treatment of fabricated illness (Goldfarb, 1998). Paediatricians and other secondary care specialists have received the most attention in the child protection literature in this respect. In comparison, relatively little focus has been directed towards the role of the general practitioner (GP) in the natural history of MSBP, a finding which is not in keeping with the significant role that GPs undertake in the provision of health care for children as well as their families. In Jamie's case, the paediatrician, like others before him, was focused almost entirely upon the symptoms as presented by his mother. It must be remembered that paediatrics is a specialty where there is an emphasis on history taking and listening to carer's concerns. The paediatrician was at a disadvantage in that he did not have available to him the full picture of the family's

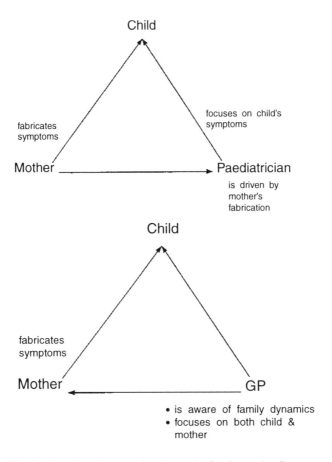

Fig. 1. Relationships in Munchausen's Syndrome by Proxy.

psycho-social dynamics while the GP, on the other hand was aware of the mother's psychiatric history. The GP at a later discussion with the paediatrician revealed that while she had considerable concerns regarding the welfare of the children in this family, she felt constrained by issues relating to confidentiality. In addition, even though she was willing to participate actively in the child protection plan, she feared that her attendance at the child protection case conference would compromise her professional relationship with Jamie's mother. Furthermore, she was aware of the controversy surrounding MSBP in both the medical journals and popular press (Fisher and Mitchell, 1995).

GPS AND CHILD HEALTH

In the United Kingdom, GPs rather than paediatricians are usually the first point of contact for child health issues which require professional opinion. In addition, GPs and health visitors are responsible for undertaking the majority of child health surveillance programmes (Gillam and Colver, 1993). As a result, they will inevitably encounter situations where they suspect child abuse or neglect. The exact prevalence of MSBP remains unknown and many consider it to be a rare phenomenon. Data which has been collected prospectively over two years by the British Paediatric Association Surveillance Unit would suggest that the combined annual incidence of MSBP, non-accidental poisoning and suffocation is 0.5/100,000 for children aged under 16 years and 2.8/100,000 for children aged under one year (McClure *et al.*, 1996). The true prevalence is probably higher as this estimate is based upon confirmed cases following extensive investigation. Hence on a national perspective, GPs and other members of the primary health care team (PHCT) will encounter children who are victims of MSBP.

There has been a demonstrable shift towards a primary care led health service in recent years, a trend which has continued since the Alma Ata conference in 1978 where it was declared that the overall goal of improving health was to be achieved through primary care (World Health Organization, 1978). Numerous attempts have been made to define the concept "primary care". The most comprehensive and that which is most descriptive of primary care within the United Kingdom has been devised by Tudor Hart (Royal College of General Practitioners, 1992):

The point where the NHS is seen as a whole and the people it serves; a close underview from where the action begins, rather than an overview from hospital specialism where some of it ends, or from the outer space of a university library.

This definition underlines the holistic nature of primary care which differs in many respects from more specialised, secondary care services. Primary care is family orientated and offers services for patients of all ages. It therefore provides for first contact, continuous comprehensive and co-ordinated care with an emphasis on disease prevention and health promotion. The importance of primary care has been strengthened by recent health care reform in the United Kingdom and in particular by the emergence of Primary Care Groups (Department of Health, 1996). No discussion of any child health issue would be complete, therefore, without a consideration of the GP's role.

Despite the importance of primary care in the promotion of children's health, relatively little is known about MSBP within the context of primary care in terms of its frequency and mode of presentation to GPs and how they might respond when they suspect that a child may be the victim of fabricated illness. Of 105 papers relating to MSBP published in peer reviewed journals within the past five years, just one made a specific reference in this context, when Ostfeld and Feldman attempted to assess the knowledge of American primary care doctors of this disorder (Ostfeld and Feldman, 1996). It was found that primary care physicians had a limited understanding of this issue. As far as we aware, no similar study has been conducted to date within the United Kingdom.

GPS AND CHILD PROTECTION

In defining a perspective from general practice upon MSBP, it might be useful to review what is already known of child protection issues in general within the context of primary care and extend this to the consideration of MSBP. GPs have been the subject of criticism because of their apparent lack of involvement in the child protection process. Despite their extensive involvement in the health of children and their ongoing contact with families, it is a fact that the majority of referrals to child protection agencies are made by professionals other than GPs (Hallett and Birchall, 1992). In the United Kingdom, the main focus of the assessment and intervention process is the child protection case conference. Here, important information regarding the child and family is shared in an attempt to assess risk and, if necessary, to define an effective child protection plan. It has been consistently observed that the majority of conferences in most districts are not attended by GPs even when adequate notice is given (Simpson *et al.*, 1994). While acknowledging the potential difficulties faced by busy GPs in attending child protection case conferences, there is an inference that their lack of participation might in part result from an unwillingness to become involved. Finally it has been shown that of all of the key professionals groups involved in the care of children, GPs receive the least amount of child protection training (Hallet, 1997). Moreover, attendance by them of child protection training events has been disappointing even when training needs analysis have been completed and accreditation for postgraduate education (PGEA) obtained (Hendry, 1997).

ATTITUDES HELD BY GPS TOWARDS THE CHILD PROTECTION PROCESS

Some insight into the background for this apparent lack of commitment by GPs to a key issue in child welfare is provided from a review of the world literature on child abuse and neglect and from recent research undertaken in the West Midlands, United Kingdom. There is a relative paucity of literature which considers the involvement of primary care doctors in the child abuse process. However, a number of papers have emphasised themes which are of relevance:

• Doctors of all backgrounds, including those who work in primary care demonstrate a reluctance to report instances of suspected abuse even in countries where reporting is mandatory (Warner and Hansen, 1994).
• Personal characteristics of doctors (i.e., age, sex, personal history of abuse, previous training on child protection) influence their behaviour when they encounter instances of suspected child abuse. The inference is that doctors who are female, younger or who have had experience of critical incidents in practice are more likely to be receptive to allegations of child abuse and to make appropriate referrals to child protection agencies (Johnson, 1993).

- The legal, moral and ethical dimensions of the GP's role in child protection work are also worthy of consideration. Confidentiality remains a powerful medical tradition and many family doctors have reservations about sharing sensitive information with statutory agencies. At the same time, others are fearful of the repercussions of not reporting instances of abuse (Halverson *et al.*, 1993).

While the above themes are descriptive of GPs' attitudes and behaviour towards child abuse work in general, they are also relevant within the context of MSBP. It may be surmised that GPs may be more reluctant to become involved in the assessment and intervention of this form of child abuse.

Further information was provided following focus group discussions on the subject of child abuse and neglect which were conducted among five primary health care teams in the West Midlands, United Kingdom (Bannon, Carter and Ross, in press). There was considerable confusion with respect to precise definition of the role of the GP in child protection work; this confusion was expressed both by the GPs themselves and by other members of the PHCT. Child protection was a source of considerable anxiety and uncertainty to GPs. This was especially the case with respect to definition of their role in child protection work, their lack of clarity with respect to referral processes and the perceived potential for damage to their relationship with families whenever they initiated child protection procedures. GPs held ambivalent views with respect to their attendance at child protection case conferences with many expressing the opinion that that they had little to contribute to the process. While acknowledging their lack of awareness of this area and expressing a wish for further training, they did not appear eager to increase their commitment to child protection work. Lack of time was frequently mentioned as a contributory factor.

GPS' TRAINING NEEDS IN CHILD PROTECTION

As professionals who work in a front-line situation with children and their families, it is possible that they may have unrecognised training needs with respect to their participation in child protection work. A postal questionnaire survey was undertaken amongst a random 10% sample of GPs in England in order to determine their perceived child protection training needs (Bannon and Carter, 1998). 1,000 GPs replied and the main training themes elicited were as follows:

1. **Detection of abuse** was by far the commonest identified category. This referred to the perceived need to develop improved standards in the prompt identification of all types of child abuse and neglect.
2. **Legal aspects** were of two categories: improved understanding of recent legislation and an appreciation of the medico-legal implications for doctors of their involvement in the child protection process.
3. **Intervention procedures** when abuse was suspected or identified included appreciation of when the threshold for intervention had been exceeded as well as local referral processes.
4. **Interagency liaison** was a broad topic which covered both an appreciation of the roles of other agencies in the child protection process (Social Services, Police, Accident and Emergency Departments) as well as means of communicating with them.
5. **Child protection case conferences** resulted in three areas of training need: (1) some GPs wished to have a greater understanding of the wider implications for them when they attended conferences (2) guidance with respect to the preparation and presentation of reports for conferences (3) how to deal with the presence of parents at conferences.
6. **Support for families** referred to an understanding of available sources and mechanisms of support for families after the intervention/investigation process had been completed.
7. **Emotional reaction** included the training required by doctors to cope with their own feelings when they encountered child abuse or neglect.

While these perceived training needs were generic to child protection issues as a whole, they are equally applicable to MSBP.

CHALLENGES FACED BY GPS

It may be concluded, therefore, that a number of separate factors (Fig. 2), working in synergy, may explain the apparent reluctance by

Imprecise role definition	Unmet training needs
Uncertainty	Impaired awareness
Anxiety	
Reluctance to become involved	

Fig. 2. Challenges faced by GPs within the context of child abuse or neglect.

family doctors to become more intimately involved in the child protection process.

- Impaired awareness of child protection issues will of necessity result from lack of training and education. Following the findings of the training needs analysis of GPs in England, it may well be the case that the content of currently available training for GPs might not accurately reflect upon their specific needs within the broad context of family medicine.
- Lack of clarity regarding their precise role in the protection of children from abuse and neglect will lead to uncertainty and lack of confidence on the part of GPs whenever they encounter situations where they suspect that child abuse or neglect has occurred.
- Anxiety is a powerful emotion which may influence the attitudes and resulting behaviour of doctors. It may be caused by uncertainty and fear of the unknown. However, fear of the legal implications for doctors who do become involved in child protection issues represents another recurring theme in the world literature (van Veenendaal, 1993). Some GPs may fear the medico-legal consequences of disclosing confidential information to social services against the expressed wishes of parents if, following investigation, no evidence of abuse is found. Others may also have concerns regarding the legal implications of not referring cases of abuse to the statutory agencies (Carter, 1995). Anxiety is also likely to arise as a result of concern that the unique relationship that GPs enjoy with families may be compromised if they become involved in child protection work. This

• Family medicine	Child protection process
• Family support	Paramountcy principle
• Confidentiality	Information sharing
• Professional autonomy	Interagency collaboration

Fig. 3.   Tensions: family medicine *versus* child protection.

represents a fundamental issue which perhaps illustrates clearly the ideological tensions that may exist between family medicine and child protection principles (Fig. 3). The philosophy of primary care is essentially orientated towards entire families and often communities. Social workers and paediatricians, while allegedly aware of the importance of family relationships and dynamics, inevitably focus their attention and decision making process upon the needs of the child. While most GPs will claim that they support the principle of child paramountcy, in practice, doing so will present them with difficulties. Respect for patient confidentiality is a guiding principle for general practice and primary care. Unfortunately, adherence to the child protection process frequently will require that sensitive information, given in confidence by patients, may need to be shared with other agencies in order to ensure the protection of children. Finally, GPs within the United Kingdom are most frequently independent, self employed practitioners who provide services by means of a contractual arrangement with health agencies. There is no absolute requirement for them to work closely with social services and follow child protection guidelines. However, from 1999, this situation is likely to change as primary care groups draw on locally formulated health improvement plans and consider how to strategically develop services for their communities. New local multidisciplinary alliances will allow professionals to work closely with patients. This will encourage collaboration between health and social services, particularly, in deprived areas where health agencies strive to reduce health inequality.

DOES THE GP HAVE A ROLE IN THE MANAGEMENT OF SUSPECTED MSBP?

The principles of the child protection process have been defined in *Working Together* (Working Together under the Children Act, 1989). In order that children remain safe from the threat of abuse or neglect, it is essential that all professionals who have significant contact with them and their families adhere to the paramountcy principle which places the welfare of children above all other consideration, that they are committed to interagency collaboration and that they work as far as possible in partnership with parents. Participation in child protection work is potentially demanding for professionals. The ultimate in clinical acumen, communication skills, problem solving and clinical decision making is necessary. Child protection procedures inevitably require some degree of confrontation with carers and furthermore, professionals must be also prepared to testify in court in order to defend their actions and views. These skills are especially relevant when professionals encounter situations where they suspect that a child may be the victim of MSBP. Most child protection experts will admit that management of suspected MSBP is fraught with difficulty; it is likely to be even more challenging for GPs. It has been argued therefore, that GPs should have a minimal role in the child protection process because of the difficulties they encounter, their current low profile in child protection work and their reluctance to become involved (Hallett, 1995). However, as Jamie's case history will demonstrate, the GP, while reluctant to become actively involved, had a key role to play by means of providing social services with valuable information and also by undertaking to provide ongoing support and treatment for Jamie's mother. The question to be addressed is whether GPs can contribute to the child protection process in a manner which does not compromise their subsequent relationships with families.

Way Forward

The child protection process may be considered from a number of viewpoints but may usefully be divided into three broad categories: detection, assessment

Elements of the child protection process	Requirements within the context of primary care
Detection: • vigilance • recognition	**Awareness of:** • clinical indicators of MSBP • local referral processes **Communication:** • within PHCT • with other agencies
Intervention: • reporting to statutory agencies • assessment of risk • definition of child protection plan	**Commitment to:** • paramountcy principle • interagency working • information sharing
Rehabilitation: • implementation of child protection plan • re-evaluation • family support • prevention of further abuse	**Involvement of GP and PHCT at each stage**

Fig. 4.   The role of the GP in the management of MSBP.

and intervention (Fig. 4). The role of the GP should be considered in terms of each of these categories.

Detection of abuse requires a combination of awareness of the clinical indicators of abuse as well as maintenance of constant vigilance. In addition there must be mechanisms whereby members of the PHCT may share concerns with each other. Difficulties arise here because as yet there is no consensus of opinion with respect to exactly what constitutes clear evidence of MSBP as it would present to primary care. In many cases of established MSBP, the GP is by-passed in favour of paediatricians and other secondary care specialists. At the same time, GPs would be rightly reluctant to label all mothers who are anxious or who present regularly with their children as perpetrators of abuse. Further work is needed to develop guidelines which would help GPs in this respect.

The next stage in the child protection process is crucial and represents the moment when concerns on the part of a doctor become "public" and are shared with outside agencies such as social services or paediatricians. It is acknowledged that GPs will find it difficult to refer families to the statutory agencies when they suspect MSBP. However, the child protection process should be flexible enough to enable them to fulfil their obligations to the safety of the child while, at the same time, as far as it is possible, allowing them to maintain their relationships with families. Confidential planning meetings have been used with success in other circumstances where complex abuse has been suspected and the same process could be employed here whereby GPs could discuss their concerns in confidence. Designated paediatricians have a specific responsibility in supporting their primary care colleagues in this respect.

The final stage is that of provision of support for the family and addressing the needs of the mother. This represents a crucial part of the process where the GP has much to offer but this can only occur if GPs have been included in the process from the beginning.

Further collaborative work is needed in order that GPs may contribute to the protection of children from fabricated illness. Child protection agencies should work closely with all those who have a responsibility for GP education and training to ensure that GPs possess an adequate awareness of this subject. Further research and debate is required in order to both define the most appropriate role that the GP and health visitor should undertake in this area as well strategies to maintain relationships with families. Continuing professional development should allow for individual lifelong learning as well as development of the practice as a learning team environment (Carter, Jackson and Barnfield, 1998). Action is also required upon the part of GPs and their teams in that they must acknowledge that they have a key role to play in ensuring that children remain safe from this most serious form of abuse.

REFERENCES

Bannon, M. J., Carter, Y. H., Ross, E. (1999). Perceived barriers to full participation by general practitioners in the child protection process: Preliminary conclusions from focus group discussions in West Midlands, UK. *J. Interprof. Care* **13**: 239–248.

Bannon, M. J., Carter, Y. H. (1998). *An Evaluation of the Training Needs of General Practitioners in England in Child Protection*. London: Queen Mary And Westfield College.

Carter, Y. H. (1995). Child Abuse: A Dilemma for General Practice. (Editorial) *Update,* January 60–61.

Carter, Y. H., Jackson, N., Barnfield, A. (1998). The learning practice: A new model for primary health care teams. *Educ. Gen. Pract.* **9**: 182–187.

Department of Health. (1996). *Primary Care: Delivering the Future*. London: HMSO.

Fisher, G. C., Mitchell, I. (1995). Is Munchausen Syndrome by Proxy really a syndrome? *Arch. Dis. Child.* **72**: 530–534.

Gillam, S. J., Colver, A. (1993). Pre-school child health surveillance. *Quality in Health Care* **2**: 129–133.

Goldfarb, J. (1998). A physician's perspective on dealing with cases of Munchausen by Proxy. *Clin. Pediatr.* **37**: 187–189.

Hallett, C., Birchall, E. (1992). *Co-ordination and Child Protection*. London: HMSO.

Hallett, C. (1995). *Inter-agency Co-ordination in Child Protection*. London: HMSO.

Halverson, K. C., Elliott, B. A., Rubin, M. S., Chadwick, D. L. (1993). Legal considerations in cases of child abuse. *Primary Care; Clinics in Office Practice* **20**: 407–416.

Hendry, E. (1997). Engaging general practitioners in child protection training. *Child Abuse Rev.* **6**: 60–64.

Johnson, C. F. (1993). Physicians and medical neglect: Variables that affect reporting. *Child Abuse Negl.* **17**: 605–612.

McClure, R. J., Davis, P. M., Meadow, S. R., Sibert, J. R. (1996). Epidemiology of Munchausen Syndrome by Proxy, non-accidental poisoning, and non-accidental suffocation. *Arch. Dis. Child.* **75**: 57–61.

Murray, J. B. (1997). Munchausen Syndrome/Munchausen Syndrome by Proxy. *J. Psychol.* **131**: 343–352.

Ostfeld, B. M., Feldman, M. D. (1996). Factitious disorder by proxy: Awareness among mental health practitioners. *Gen. Hosp. Psychiatry* **18**: 113–116.

Royal College of General Practitioners. (1992). *Forty Years On. The Story of the First Forty Years of the Royal College of General Practitioners.* London: Royal College of General Practitioners.

Simpson, C. M., Simpson, R. J., Power, K. G., Salter, A., Williams, G. (1994). GPs' and health visitors' participation in child protection case conferences. *Child Abuse Rev.* **3**: 211–230.

van Veenendaal, E. (1993). Child abuse: Does disclosing the fact have implications for medical secrecy? *Med. Law* **12**: 25–28.

Warner, J. E., Hansen, D. J. (1994). The identification and reporting of physical abuse by physicians: A review and implications for research. *Child Abuse Negl.* **18**: 11–25.

World Health Organization. (1978). *Primary Health Care.* Geneva.

Working Together under the Children Act 1989. HMSO: London.

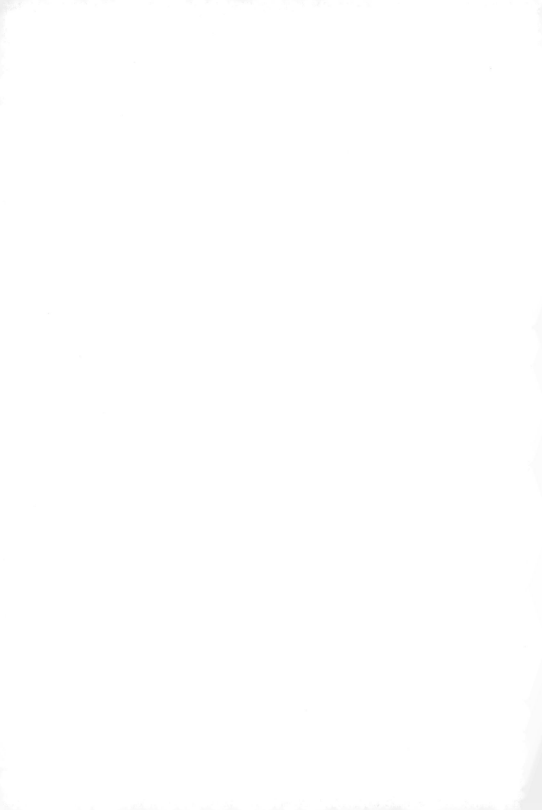

CHAPTER 6

The Presentation and Natural History of Munchausen Syndrome by Proxy

MICHAEL C.B. PLUNKETT
Specialist Registrar in Paediatrics

DAVID P. SOUTHALL
*Consultant Paediatrician/Professor of Paediatrics and
Director of Child Advocacy International,
Academic Department of Paediatrics,
North Staffordshire Hospital*

An understanding of factitious illness (Munchausen Syndrome by Proxy) requires that we are able to recognise how it may present and the course it may follow if allowed to go unchecked. Before trying to identify these features, we need to accept that this diagnostic entity exists and be prepared to entertain the diagnosis when the typical features present. Its recognition is difficult, but possible, if we allow ourselves to consider that the ill-fitting pattern of history, symptoms and signs that is presented may be a construct designed to fool medical and nursing staff.

It is also essential to be able to recognise the presentations (and natural histories) of the wide range of "natural illnesses" and remember that it is normal that when children become unwell (or are thought to be unwell) parents become anxious, seeking reassurance, telling the truth as they see or experience it. Not uncommonly, this may lead them to exaggerate or even invent symptoms. It is important that these normal parents are offered the necessary support and reassurance in a way that does not threaten the doctor–parent relationship.

PRESENTATION OF MUNCHAUSEN SYNDROME BY PROXY

In the majority of significant disease processes, even when the diagnosis is unclear, presentation of the disease is followed by attempts to define the illness and alleviate the symptoms and thus interrupt or alter the natural history. With factitious illness, the initial presentation, the investigations and any treatment (indeed any involvement of the doctor) all become part of the natural history of this most unnatural illness, as does any re-presentation and subsequent medical involvement. The natural history continues to unfold until the diagnosis is recognised and adequate protection of the child procured. Significant previous medical involvement (before the diagnosis is recognised) may affect clinical objectivity as we deal with our own (or our colleague's) prior, unwitting participation in the disease process.

The medical model of illness, demanding a treatment based on symptoms and signs supported by investigations, serves doctors and children well in dealing with natural disease processes. When the symptoms and signs are fabricated or induced and the investigations wilfully obfuscated or manipulated, what remains is a devious construct which will fool those doctors who refuse to entertain the diagnosis of factitious illness, and which may damage or kill the child.

Warning signals may alert the clinician to the possibility that the presenting symptoms have been fabricated. These signals may be viewed as clinical alerts rather than a profile of the abuser. Either way they may help the clinician to discriminate between abusive and normal parents and thus avoid complicity in the parental abuse. These clinical alerts (see Table 1), initially described by Meadow (Meadow, 1985) have been added to subsequently (Gale and Horner, 1992; Rosen et al., 1983; Eminson and Postlethwaite, 1992; Warner and Hathaway, 1984 and Southall et al., 1997), but need not be regarded as definitive.

The majority of presentations are as acute medical problems. Presenting features or symptoms affect most systems (see Table 2). In all, over 100 different symptoms have been reported (Rosenberg, 1987). The nature of this disorder is such that no list can be conclusive and the list provided here is simply for descriptive purposes, indicating the range of reported symptoms and positively identified causes.

Table 1.   Warning signals that might alert a clinician to the presence of a factitious illness.

In the child

- Illness (or signs and reported symptoms) that defy explanation leading experienced clinicians to remark that they have not seen the like of it before.
- Symptoms and signs that start only when a particular carer (usually the mother) is present.
- Symptoms and signs that resolve spontaneously (or do not recur) when the child is separated from a particular carer.
- Multiple physician involvement in child's management.
- Treatments that are unexpectedly ineffective or poorly tolerated.

In the child's history

- Reported symptoms which may be unverifiable.
- Multiple hospitalisations experienced by child.
- Alleged allergies to a great variety of foods and drugs.
- Serious illnesses claimed to have been identified at other hospitals.
- Complex pattern of previous medical care hidden by carer from the paediatrician.
- Inconsistencies between carer's historical accounts and clinical/laboratory findings of recognisable diseases.
- Apparent life-threatening events associated with bleeding from the nose or mouth.

In the family history

- Families in which unexplained infant deaths have occurred.
- Families in which many members are alleged to have different serious medical disorders.
- Families with a history of unexplained infant death or unexplained apparent life-threatening events associated with bleeding from the nose or mouth.

In the carer

- Other carer typically uninvolved in the care of the child.
- Carers who have (or falsely claim to have) medical (or nursing/paramedical) knowledge or training.
- Carers who are not as concerned by the child's illness as the medical and nursing staff, who remain with the child constantly or who are happily at ease on the children's ward, forming unusually close relationships with the staff.
- Carers who have invested significant emotional/intellectual effort in the illness. This may be exhibited in their involvement in self-help and activist groups and subsequent courting of press publicity, where the illness becomes part of their identity.
- Carers who have a history of conduct or eating disorders.
- Carers who have a history of unusual illness (which may be unverifiable) or themselves have suffered or give a history of physical, emotional or sexual abuse in childhood.
- Carers who have Munchausen Syndrome or somatisation disorder.

Table 2. Presentations (symptoms, signs and diseases) that have been reported in Munchausen Syndrome by Proxy, and their causes (where positively identified).

System	Symptom/Sign/Disease	Cause
Neurological	Seizures, collapse and loss of consciousness, ataxia, drowsiness; developmental delay, deafness	Drugs (Southall et al., 1997; Rogers, 1976 and Waller, 1983), poisons (Southall et al., 1997 and Hickson et al., 1989), suffocation (Southall et al., 1997; Mitchell et al., 1993; Alexander et al., 1990 and Meadow, 1998), pressure on carotid sinus (Meadow, 1982)
Cardiorespiratory	Apnoeic and cyanotic episodes, cardiac arrest, "near-miss SIDS"	Suffocation with hands, cloth, plastic bag or film (Rosen et al., 1983; Southall et al., 1987; Southall et al., 1997; Boros et al., 1995; Alexander et al., 1990; Meadow, 1990; Berger, 1979 and Hickson et al., 1989)
	Cystic fibrosis	Altering laboratory investigations and stealing sputum from other patients (Orenstein et al., 1986)
	Asthma	Deliberate under/over treatment (Godding and Kruth, 1991 and Masterson et al., 1988)
Gastrointestinal	Recurrent vomiting and diarrhoea	Drugs, poisons (Epstein et al., 1987, McGuire and Feldman, 1989 and Fleischer and Ament, 1977) or mechanically induced (Alexander et al., 1990)
	Failure to thrive	Restricting intake (Warner and Hathaway, 1984), altering intravenous infusion, aspirating nasogastric tube (Southall et al., 1997; McGuire and Feldman, 1989; Alexander et al., 1990 and Roesler et al., 1994)

Table 2.   *(Continued)*

System	Symptom/Sign/Disease	Cause
Renal	Polyuria, polydipsia	Drugs (Verity *et al.*, 1979)
	Haematuria, renal stone	Adding stone, parental blood and colouring substances to urine (Meadow, 1977)
	Bacteruria	Swapping urine specimens with parent or other patients (Meadow, 1977)
Haematological	Purpura	Injecting blood under skin, rubbing skin (Meadow, 1982)
	Haematemesis, haemoptysis and rectal bleeding	Adding parental blood to specimens, clothing and nappies (McGuire and Feldman, 1989; Alexander *et al.*, 1990; Meadow, 1998 and Berger, 1979)
Immunological	Recurrent fever, sepsis	Heating thermometer (Meadow, 1982), injecting bacteriologically contaminated material, interfering with intravenous sites (Boros *et al.*, 1995 and Kohl *et al.*, 1978)
	Allergy	Applying excessive environmental and dietary measures to avoid "allergen" (Warner and Hathaway, 1984 and Roesler *et al.*, 1994)
Dermatological	Rashes	Applying irritants, scratching or injecting the skin (Southall *et al.*, 1997; Meadow, 1982 and Magnay *et al.*, 1994)
Metabolic	Hypoglycaemia, glycosuria	Abuse of insulin and sugar solutions (Verity *et al.*, 1979 and McGuire and Feldman, 1989), drugs (Rogers *et al.*, 1976)
	Hypernatraemia	Adding salt to feeds (Southall *et al.*, 1997; Meadow, 1977; Meadow, 1993b and Rogers *et al.*, 1976)

Some of the symptoms listed have been fabricated, others have been induced. Some presentations involve both fabricated history and induced illness (e.g., involving suffocation or poisoning) (McClure *et al.*, 1996). When witnessed (Southall *et al.*, 1997) the abuse has been seen to be premeditated, inflicted without provocation and appeared at times sadistic. That the fabrication and illness induction (including life-threatening abuse) has been shown to occur on children's wards, while the children were being monitored in a caring, protective environment, is evidence of its insidious nature. Explanations have often involved quite plausible lies.

The presenting symptoms may be determined by the age of the child — different forms of abuse are seen in different age groups. Apnoeic or cyanotic attacks caused by suffocation are readily produced in infants and young children. When presenting with apparent life-threatening events requiring resuscitation, infants subject to factitious illness are older (at time of first event) and less likely to be premature than infants who have a "natural" disease responsible for the events (Southall *et al.*, 1997). False allegations of physical and sexual abuse — made by the mother in respect of her child and usually in conjunction with other fabricated illness — tend to involve older children and may occur at the time of contested divorce and custody disputes (Meadow, 1993a).

NATURAL HISTORY OF MUNCHAUSEN SYNDROME BY PROXY

The natural history of Munchausen Syndrome by Proxy is both determined by and a determinant of the investigation and treatment of the presenting symptoms and signs. Thus, subsequent presentation is dependent on the medical management of the child. It can therefore be seen that a "specialised, investigation-orientated" medical system (Donald and Jureidini, 1996) encourages and supports abuse in predisposed parents. The natural history of this disorder varies from one child to another. It may be thought of as being analogous to the outcome for the child, but any understanding of that outcome must clearly recognise the suffering the child has endured, often over some considerable time (Southall *et al.*, 1997; Bools, Neale and

Meadow, 1993; Godding and Kruth, 1991 and Davis *et al.*, 1998). There are many sources that inform about the natural history of this disorder. We can examine the histories of children diagnosed as being subjected to factitious illness who have then been adequately protected form further abuse. We can look carefully at their siblings for indicators of the same abuse and re-examine the histories of any unexplained child deaths in their families. We may unfortunately be given the opportunity to re-examine victims who continue to reside with their abusing mother as they experience further fabrications or induced illness (Bools, Neale and Meadow, 1993).

Meadow (Meadow, 1989) suggests a useful method for examining the main consequences for children subjected to factitious illness.

(a) They will receive needless and harmful investigations and treatments, all prescribed, initiated or undertaken by paediatricians. From the earliest reports (Meadow, 1997), detailed accounts of unnecessary blood and radiological investigations have been cited. Treatment with anti-epileptic drugs — with or without abnormality on EEG — is common (Rosen, 1983; Southall *et al.*, 1987 and Verity *et al.*, 1979). Investigations under anaesthesia including urological examination (Meadow, 1997), open lung biopsy (Boros *et al.*, 1995), insertion of cardiac pacemaker (Rosen, 1983 and Mitchell *et al.*, 1993), insertion of central venous lines for intravenous feeding (Epstein *et al.*, 1987) and major operations such as fundoplication (Rosen, 1983; McGuire and Feldman, 1989 and Alexander *et al.*, 1990) represent an incomplete list of procedures that are not without hazard.

(b) A genuine disease or injury may be induced by the mother's actions. These may be transient and self-limiting, albeit significant conditions, such as fractures (Southall *et al.*, 1987; Mitchell *et al.*, 1993; Bryk and Siegel, 1997 and Meadow, 1998), cardiomyopathy (Goebel *et al.*, 1993) and seizures (Southall *et al.*, 1997). They may impair the quality or quantity of life in the long term such as significant behaviour problems (Southall *et al.*, 1997; Bools *et al.*, 1993 and McGuire and Feldman, 1989), "brain damage" (Southall *et al.*, 1997; Alexander *et al.*, 1990 and Meadow, 1990), spastic quadriplegia (Bools *et al.*, 1993), blindness (Southall *et al.*, 1997), pulmonary oedema requiring ventilation, leaving significant lung damage and a need for home oxygen therapy (Southall *et al.*, 1997), restrictive lung disease and growth retardation from oral steroids (Godding and Kruth, 1991).

(c) Children may die suddenly, as a result of mother misjudging the degree of insult, or deliberately, to obtain the attention that inevitably accompanies a child's death. This is more likely when the abuse involves inducing symptoms, which of themselves require life-saving treatment, rather than symptoms that may simply be indicators of life-threatening disease. Thus, provoking a convulsion by suffocation is dangerous (although epilepsy need not be) whereas presenting a child with a purpuric rash may not be intrinsically harmful, but meningococcal septicaemia is life-threatening. Mothers who denied murderous intent but who nonetheless suffocated their babies may have been trying to induce apparent life-threatening events without initially understanding just how life-threatening their actions were. Whatever the underlying intent, smothering as a means of illness induction has often proved fatal (Rosen, 1983; Southall *et al.*, 1997; Mitchell *et al.*, 1993; Alexander *et al.*, 1990; Meadow, 1998; Berger, 1979 and Meadow, 1999). It presents a particular problem for paediatricians (responsible for child protection) and pathologists (charged with determining the cause of death) as the post-mortem appearances are usually indistinguishable from naturally occurring, unexplained infant death (Meadow, 1999). That death is a common outcome in infants presenting with apparent life-threatening events caused by suffocation, can be inferred from the high incidence of unexplained infant death among siblings of infants so abused (Southall *et al.*, 1997 and Meadow, 1999). During their final hours, smothered infants have usually been observed by other adults to be well (Meadow, 1999). Salt ingestion has also frequently prove fatal (Godding and Kruth, 1991; Meadow, 1977; Meadow, 1993b and Rogers *et al.*, 1976), possibly a surprise to the parent who might have regarded it as an innocuous condiment.

(d) They may develop chronic invalidism. The child accepts the "illness story" that he has been told for so long and believes himself to be disabled and, for example, unable to attend school (Warner and Hathaway, 1984; Meadow, 1988 and Masterson *et al.*, 1988). The fabricated history or the induced illness may have led to frequent or prolonged hospitalisation for investigations and treatments resulting in literally years of school absence. The child may persist with, for example, the exaggeration of his asthmatic symptoms (Masterson *et al.*, 1988) and severe allergen avoidance measures (Warner and Hathaway, 1984) or may continue to over- or undertreat his asthma (Godding and Kruth, 1991) thus imposing or accepting significant limitations on schooling, exercise and lifestyle.

(e) They may continue to fabricate symptoms as an adult — the children have learnt and then taken over the lying behaviour of the mother, for example, persisting with the mother's assertion of headaches and fits (Bools *et al.*, 1993). Conversion disorder with blindness and paralysis has been described in adolescents previously subjected to Munchausen Syndrome by Proxy (McGuire and Feldman, 1989).

Predicting what might become of a child if the diagnosis were not realised and the child adequately protected, is difficult. Careful attention to the family history may reveal that previous siblings presented with similar symptoms. Re-examination of previous deaths in siblings may reveal them to have been "unnatural". In families where children have been subjected serially to Munchausen Syndrome by Proxy, it has been demonstrated that the abuse and the manner in which it presents is often similar and the child has a greater likelihood of being killed (Alexander *et al.*, 1990). Suffocation seems particularly common in serial abusers (Southall *et al.*, 1997; Mitchell *et al.*, 1993; Alexander *et al.*, 1990; Meadow, 1990 and Hickson *et al.*, 1989). Poisoning (Southall *et al.*, 1997 and Hickson *et al.*, 1989), sometimes with the same substance, for example, arsenic (Alexander *et al.*, 1990), or salt (Meadow, 1993) has been repeated within families as have false allegations of physical or sexual abuse (Meadow, 1993b), and fabricated histories of food allergy (Roesler *et al.*, 1994) or epilepsy (Meadow, 1998).

Finally, the purpose of understanding the presentation and natural history of Munchausen Syndrome by Proxy is to use the knowledge to protect victims and their siblings, including those not yet born, who may be viewed as potential victims. Making the diagnosis without adequately protecting the child may not significantly alter the natural history. However, one consequence of a parent's assiduous pursuit and consumption of medical attention for their child is that this natural history may be very carefully logged and available later to someone willing to entertain what previously may have seemed like an unbelievable diagnosis.

REFERENCES

Alexander, R., Smith, W., Stevenson, R. (1990). *Pediatrics* **86**: 581–585.

Berger, D. (1979). *J. Pediatr.* **95**: 554–556.

Bools, C. N., Neale, B. A., Meadow, S. R. (1993). *Arch. Dis. Child.* **69**: 625–630.

Boros, S. J., Ophoven, J. P., Anderson, R., Brubaker, L. C. (1995). *Austral. Fam. Psych.* **24**: 768–773.

Bryk, M., Siegel, P. T. (1997). *Pediatrics* **100**: 1–7.

Davis, P., *et al.* (1998). *Arch. Dis. Child.* **78**: 217–221.

Donald, T., Jureidini, J. (1996). *Arch. Pediatr. Adolesc. Med.* **150**: 753–758.

Eminson, D. M., Postlethwaite, R. J. (1992). *Arch. Dis. Child.* **67**: 1510–1516.

Epstein, M. A., *et al.* (1987). *Pediatrics* **80**: 220–224.

Fleischer, D., Ament, M. E. (1977). *Clin. Pediatr.* **17**: 820–824.

Gale, C. A., Horner, M. M. (1992). *J. Clin. Nurs.* **1**: 27–32.

Godding, V., Kruth, M. (1991). *Arch. Dis. Child.* **66**: 956–960.

Goebel, J., Gremse, D. A., Artman, M. (1993). *Pediatrics* **92**: 601–603.

Hickson, G. B., Altemeier, W. A., Martin, E. D., Campbell, P. W. (1989). *Pediatrics* **83**: 772–776.

Kohl, S., Pickering, L. K., Duprees, E. (1978). *J. Pediatr.* **95**: 466–468.

Magnay, A. R., Debelle, G., Proops, D. W., Booth, I. W. (1994). *J. Laryngol. Otol.* **108**: 336–338.

Masterson, J., Dunworth, R., Williams, N. (1988). *Amer. J. Orthopsychiat.* **58**: 188–195.

McClure, R. J., Davis, P. M., Meadow, S. R., Sibert, J. R. (1996). *Arch. Dis. Child.* **75**: 57–61.

McGuire, T. L., Feldman, K. W. (1989). *Pediatrics* **83**: 289–292.

Meadow, R. (1977). *Lancet* **2**: 343–345.

Meadow, R. (1982). *Arch. Dis. Child.* **57**: 92–98.

Meadow, R. (1985). *Arch. Dis. Child.* **60**: 385–393.

Meadow, R. (1989). *Br. Med. J.* **299**: 248–250.

Meadow, R. (1990). *J. Pediatr.* **117**: 351–357.

Meadow, R. (1993a). *Arch. Dis. Child.* **68**: 444–447.

Meadow, R. (1993b). *Arch. Dis. Child.* **68**: 448–452.

Meadow, R. (1998). *Arch. Dis. Child.* **78**: 210–216.

Meadow, R. (1999). *Arch. Dis. Child.* **80**: 7–14.

Mitchell, I., Brummitt, J., DeForest, J., Fisher, G. (1993). *Pediatrics* **92**: 810–814.

Orenstein, D. M., Wasserman, A. L. (1986). *Pediatrics* **78**: 621–624.

Roesler, T. A., Barry, P. C., Bock, A. (1994). *Arch. Pediatr. Adolesc. Med.* **148**: 1150–1155.

Rogers, D., *et al.* (1976). *Br. Med. J.* **1**: 793–796.

Rosen, C. L., *et al.* (1983). *Pediatrics* **71**: 715–720.

Rosen, C. L., Frost, J. D., Glaze, G. D. (1986). *J. Pediatr.* **109**: 1065–1067.

Rosenberg, D. A. (1987). *Child Abuse Negl.* **18**: 773–788.

Southall, D. P., *et al.* (1987). *Br. Med. J.* **294**: 1637–1641.

Southall, D. P., *et al.* (1997). *Pediatrics* **100**: 735–760.

Verity, C. M., *et al.* (1979). *Br. Med. J.* **2**: 422.

Waller, D. A. (1983). *J. Am. Acad. Child Psychol.* **22**: 80–85.

Warner, J. O., Hathaway, M. J. (1984). *Arch. Dis. Child.* **59**: 151–156.

CHAPTER 7

The Detection of Munchausen Syndrome by Proxy

MARTIN P. SAMUELS
Consultant Paediatrician/Senior Lecturer in Paediatrics,
Academic Department of Paediatrics,
North Staffordshire Hospital

The diagnosis of factitious illness (Munchausen Syndrome by Proxy) is neither straightforward nor reached quickly. It has to be actively thought about as a diagnostic possibility to explain the child's symptoms or illness, and an active approach taken to confirm the diagnosis, that is, it is not a diagnosis of exclusion (Rogers *et al.*, 1976; Meadow, 1985; Rosenberg, 1987; Jones, 1998). The diagnosis describes the clinical presentation of a child whose symptoms are either false reports by a parent or carer, or due to illness caused by them. This presentation involves exaggeration, misrepresentation, false information and deceit by a carer of the child, usually the mother, in order that they receive attention or maintain a sick role (Eminson and Postlethwaite, 1992). Because this clinical presentation involves a parent who has some disorder of personality or social functioning (Bools, Neal and Meadow, 1994), the detection involves a variety of measures to clarify objectively the presence and cause of reported symptoms and signs. In part, this may be considered good clinical practice by ensuring that investigations and treatments are targeted appropriately. However, compared to clinical practice, a more critical assessment of the child's illness is required. This is because clinicians have, firstly, to counteract the deception that accompanies factitious illness, and secondly, to provide sufficient evidence for the diagnosis to stand up in the child protection arena. This particularly applies where statutory intervention or cross-examination in a court of law are required.

A large proportion of factitious illness in paediatric practice presents in the acute sector, that is, the hospital (McClure, Davies, Meadow and Silbert, 1996). This is because alarming and frequently reported symptoms or severe illness will often necessitate hospital attendance or admission. It may be that with the increasing recognition of this condition, less severe forms of factitious illness may present in the community setting. The increasing tendency for health care to be provided in the community may also shift the presentation of fabricated illness outside of the hospital setting.

There are several reasons why it is important to detect factitious illness, mostly relating to the harm the child is subjected to (Rosenberg, 1987; Jones and Lynch, 1998; Lobow, 1995; Davis *et al.*, 1998). This harm results from (i) the physical discomfort, pain and emotional trauma that results if illness is induced (as opposed to fabricated reports of illness). The harm may occur from physical assault (e.g., attempted suffocation), poisoning or other signs produced in the child (e.g., bruising); (ii) the psychological trauma from being considered ill or handicapped, or inappropriately more so than would be expected for any true illness or condition the child does suffer from; (iii) the physical and emotional suffering as a result of unnecessary or inappropriate investigations, medication and surgical procedures, and the risks associated with these; (iv) the emotional harm which accompanies illness fabrication, as a result of the disordered relationship between parent and child — this may have long term consequences, including educational, social and occupational difficulties, low self-esteem, self-harm, illness induction and suicide attempts (Libow, 1995; Bryk and Siegel, 1997).

Failure to detect factitious illness may have professional consequences too, with clinical mysteries or challenges wasting the time of clinicians and nursing staff, and consuming resources in unnecessary investigations or treatments. Inappropriate use of such human and financial resources diverts them from other children. An active approach to confirming the diagnosis is also important, because where the suspicion of factitious illness has been raised and child protection procedures set in motion, inadequate evidence of fabrication can result in lengthy legal procedures and court time with significant additional implications for social services and legal aid resources. Finally, failure to document illness fabrication or induction with the best possible evidence can mean truthful parents themselves may suffer immense emotional trauma from allegations that may be ill-founded and unsupported (Feldman and Allen, 1996).

Donald and Jureidini aptly stated that a "medical system that is specialised, investigation-oriented, fascinated by rare conditions, often ignorant of abusive behaviours, and too accepting of reported histories" contributes to the evolution of factitious illness (Donald and Jureidini, 1996). There is concern that with increasing sub-specialisation in medical practice, the environment is increasingly created in which factitious illness situations can thrive. Although it is important to objectively verify reported symptoms and signs, over reliance on investigations may mislead and produce pitfalls which lead to the failure to detect factitious illness. The critical approach that nowadays is so much part of evidence based medicine, is a useful part of clinical practice to help in a diagnosis. The clinician who repeatedly questions the validity of reported illness, asks why symptoms or illness may be occurring, and applies this to the context in which the child presents is more likely to detect and recognise induced or fabricated illness. All clinicians working with children, including sub-specialists, will see and should recognise illness fabrication, as it may well co-exist with organic illness (Eminson and Postlewaite, 1992; Masterson, Dunworth and Williams, 1988; Godding and Kruth, 1991).

There are a number of obstacles to effective management of cases of factitious illness and it is worth being aware of these when assessing and managing cases. These obstacles are discussed in detail by Waller, 1983:

(i) focusing on the harm caused by medical investigations (Meadow, 1982), may be misplaced — the emotional and physical abuse the child may suffer as a result of the parent's behaviour are far more concerning (McGuire and Feldman, 1989; Bools, Neal and Meadow, 1992), and as with any potential child protection issue, this requires a multi-agency approach to investigation (i.e., not just medical).

(ii) the parent suspected of fabrication may give the appearance of being such a trustful, caring and concerned parent that it can make it difficult for health and social service professionals to believe abuse is occurring.

(iii) the usual response of the parent to any confrontation is denial, with or without hostility. This denial makes working together with the parents difficult for health professionals and social services and may explain why there may be reluctance sometimes to entertain this diagnosis in the first place (Siegel, 1998). The parent may also be able to obtain support for her position from relatives, non-medical professionals (e.g., clergy) and health professionals (e.g., health visitor, general practitioner) who have seen her as a caring parent. The denial of fabricated illness by the mother is a prime reason for ensuring the evidence upon which the diagnosis is based is optimal: mothers have even denied attempted suffocation of their infant despite the presence of video evidence (Samuels *et al.*, 1992). A well defended denial of illness induction can be dangerous, as children have been removed by the suspected parent from the hospital setting, only to suffer subsequent sudden death (Waller, 1983; Meadow, 1990).

(iv) the abusing parent may appear so pausible that lawyers and judges may fail to understand how the parent can simultaneously be seeking medical care, and falsely reporting or inducing illness in the child. This pattern of deceit may continue so that psychiatrists involved with the child or parent may also be mislead into believing, for example, the mother has only short term difficulties or has responded to therapy. Any long term follow-up should involve health professionals and social services who communicate well and can corroborate from sources independent of the family any progress that has been made. Jucidial findings of fact in cases of fabricated illness may help reduce the "inevitable scepticism that creeps into these cases as time goes on" (Waller, 1983).

Previous reviews have discussed strategies that help in the diagnosis (Rogers *et al.*, 1976; Meadow, 1987; Rosenberg, 1987). There follows further discussion of the methods used to detect illness fabrication or induction in a child (see Table 1).

Table 1.   Methods for confirming MSBP.

History	— obtain reports from independent witnesses for symptoms/signs of illness — verify details of reported personal, social and family history — check illness history of siblings and parents with GP/other hospitals — consider motivation/gain obtained by illness behaviour
Examination	— complete and forensic in approach (consider signs of other abuse)
Observations	— for in-patients: nurse (not parent) records all observed (versus reported) symptoms/signs — one-to-one nursing observation — record all parent visits and activities with child for temporal associations
Investigations	— forensic process for collection of specimens — analysis of source and identity (patient, mother, other) of specimen — toxicology screening (consider use of police forensic laboratory) — obtain video records of symptoms and signs — physiological (event) recordings (cardiomemo, multi-channel respiratory or neurophysiological recordings) — covert video surveillance
Management	— provide parents with letter for open access to admission unit to confirm reported symptoms — stop medications/observe/document baseline investigations — food or substance challenges (double blind) — one-to-one nursing — exclusion of parents (voluntarily or by statutory intervention) — professionals strategy meeting (chaired by social services) — child protection investigation — confrontation (beware in illness induction)

THE HISTORY

As with other forms of child abuse, it is important that the history is taken ensuring full details are obtained of the reported symptoms. For fabricated reports of illness, it is the history that may be most likely to indicate a problem with illness perception or behaviour in the parent. There needs to be an examination of the internal consistency of the history with regard to timing, witnesses and situations of reported symptoms. The doctor needs to have a view as to the likely physical validity of the symptoms. It may be that the paediatrician needs to discuss the likelihood that symptoms or events have occurred as reported with either a colleague or a sub-specialist. For example, in a reported cyanotic episode, is it likely that the mother's report of cardiac arrest at home for four minutes is true? (It is of course possible that such physiological inconsistencies are simply due to innocent misperceptions.)

It is worth asking about who else witnessed the reported symptoms. Without showing disbelief and at this stage threatening the parent–doctor relationship, it is useful to obtain a separate story from these individuals. This may be the other parent, friend or relative. It is important to be aware that their reports may be coloured by false information fed to them by the parent fabricating the report. More objective and independent reports may be obtained from the child's school, nursery or minder.

Often the reported history may include details of past medical history including previous hospital admissions, investigations and treatment. Details of these should be cross checked with the relevant clinicians and copies of medical records sought for previously reported historical details, clinical findings, results of investigations, etc. Illness fabrication may not be new, but may have gone previously unnoticed. Telephone contact with clinicians previously involved with the patient and his/her family may help identify concerns that had previously been considered, but not written in the case notes or correspondence.

A reported drug history may be checked by the collection of blood or urine for confirmation that there is drug compliance. At the same time this may help in excluding drug toxicity from prescribed or other medications. In addition, if there are, for example, neurological or gastrointestinal symptoms not readily explained by organic pathology, such specimens may help identify medicines or toxins given to induce such illness. In considering poisoning, it is useful to know the drugs available at home and the employment of the parents (Rogers *et al.*, 1976).

A thorough family history should be collected particularly with regard to the parent or carer suspected of fabricating illness. Often they suffer from abnormal illness behaviour, ranging from hypochondriasis, through somatoform disorder to Munchausen Syndrome. Distinctions between these patterns of behaviour relate to the severity of the disease(s) and the degree of conscious motivation that leads to their production. It is usually not easy to determine the motivation for fabricating illness, and the degree of awareness in the parent. An extensive past medical history in the mother can usually be cross checked against her own hospital medical records (including obstetric), or with the general practitioner records, or both (Bools *et al.*, 1994; Jureidini, 1993). Sometimes, the mother may not report extensive medical consultation, and therefore it is still worthwhile undertaking a review of these records. Although consent for such an examination may be sought on the grounds that there may be a link between the child's unexplained illness and previous family illnesses, this form of preliminary investigation can be undertaken without consent for the purposes of assessing whether child protection concerns exist (Social Services Inspectorate, 1994).

A high proportion of published cases of factitious illness have reported co-morbidity in siblings (McClure *et al.*, 1996; Smith and Stevenson, 1990), and it is therefore important to document their medical histories and attendances at hospitals and, in addition examine their medical records. It is worth asking about pets in the home and their well-being. There are often features of a disorder of personality in the parent (Bools *et al.*, 1994), particularly in one who induces illness, and it can be of value to ask about any other problems at home (e.g., burglaries, arson), and the involvement of the police.

One of the main problems with the collection of historical details from the parent suspected of fabricating illness lies in the ability to collect a truthful account of the facts. Such parents misrepresent, mislead and give either exaggerated or false information. As doctors, we are trained to trust in the information the parents of our patients supply us with. However, having a degree of scepticism helps keep objectivity — thus we must listen to parents, and then consider whether their account is firstly, likely to be consistent with physical illness, and secondly, truthful. Parents who have not been readily reassured about their child's well being may also be indicating their need to maintain a sick role. The demeanour of the parent giving the history may point to problems, for example, if they appear emotionally flat, lack eye contact, or are surprisingly calm about symptoms that would concern most parents. The parent's morphology may also be important, with extremes of weight (anorexia, obesity) indicating a possible associated eating disorder.

THE EXAMINATION

As with any potential child protection case, a full medical examination must be performed and documented. Measurement of height and weight should be plotted along with any previous measurements available, as previously unrecognised failure to thrive or growth failure may be found (Bools *et al.*, 1992). The child's demeanour should be noted, for example, it would be unusual for clinicians to see obviously sad and dejected looking children. If this is observed, it may indicate abuse and should be compared with the views of other professionals who have been involved with the child. It is important to note the interaction between parent and child, whether the child freely seeks comfort from the parent and whether the parent gives an appropriate balance of positive and controlling comments to the child. Overt or harsh criticism without praise and encouragement may indicate emotional abuse.

A gross physical examination should be undertaken to look for any injury, including a search for the usual stigmata of physical abuse, such as bony lumps indicative of healing fractures, torn frenulum, retinal haemorrhages, genital injuries, and skin markings such as bites, pinches, cigarette burns, etc. The finding of fresh blood, excoriations or ulcers at a body orifice should prompt consideration that trauma may have occurred (Magnay *et al.*, 1994; Southall *et al.*, 1997).

INVESTIGATIONS

For fabricated reports of illness, investigations may do little to definitively refute or confirm the reported observations, and may in fact confuse the picture. For example, a child with fabricated reports of fits can have abnormal epileptiform discharges on EEG without this necessarily confirming that all reported fits actually happened and were organic in origin. Similarly, positive skin prick or IgE RASTs tests does not necessarily imply that symptoms were definitely due to the reported food allergy (Warner and Hatherway, 1984; Roesler *et al.*, 1994). The specificity of most investigations is well below 100%. Furthermore, because of the lack of data on large normal populations, abnormal investigation results in symptomatic children are probably more likely to be attributed as significant and the cause of reported symptoms. Some abnormal investigations may have been caused by abuse, for example, EEG slowing in encephalopathy from suffocation or poisoning. It is important that clinicians treat the child, and not simply the abnormal test results. For example, an abnormal oesophageal pH study is not necessarily the cause of recurrent apnoea — it may be the result of respiratory illness, or even coincidental with attempted suffocation by a parent.

Confirmation of fabrication of infrequent reported symptoms is problematic, and the most suitable management strategy may be to limit investigations and treatments. If a parent has reported an infrequent, but sufficiently prolonged symptom, it may be possible to supply them with a letter giving them immediate access to the admission unit or ward where a further report of the symptoms can be collected along with any supportive findings on examination. Relevant investigations may be collected such as swabs, urine specimens (e.g., for infection, or toxicology if poisoning suspected), etc. It is common that with this offer, the reported symptoms seem to abate, or the parent is unable for a variety of reasons to bring their child for attendance and examination. Withholding investigations and treatments until the child is seen in hospital when symptomatic, will avoid unnecessary treatment for infrequent fabricated symptoms.

Another method for obtaining a record confirming the reported symptoms is to ask the parent to make a video record. Many families either own or have access to video recorders. Alternatively, it should be possible for all paediatric departments to have access to such equipment specifically for the purpose of recording intermittent or unusual symptoms. Such equipment can also serve other purposes, such as providing a record of organic phenomena for the opinion of sub-specialists, or for educational purposes.

As well as video recordings, it is possible to undertake physiological recordings in a home setting (Poets *et al.*, 1993). This is particularly useful for episodes or events which would be expected to involve a change in cardiorespiratory or neurophysiological variables. For suspected arrhythmias, patients can be supplied with a cardiomemo which is placed on the chest at the time of reported symptoms, and records heart rhythm. Unfortunately, no similar device is available for such rapid EEG or respiratory recordings. For colour changes in a child, it is possible to apply pulse oximeters with internal memories, but interpretation of these should be made carefully, ensuring that adequate pulse detection has occurred, as it is possible for these machines to be interfered with in such a way that false readings are obtained. Continuous tape recordings may be made of EEG or electrocardiogram (ECG), but for infrequent events, such recordings may not be practical. Event recordings using digital memory cards have been made in young children and infants and have been able to confirm both organic and non-organic pathology (Poets *et al.*, 1993). The latter has included both fabrication of apnoeic attacks, including interfering with monitoring equipment, and actual induction of illness through imposed upper airway obstruction (Samuels *et al.*, 1992; Southall *et al.*, 1997).

For frequently reported symptoms, the simplest method for confirming their validity would be to provide a period of hospital admission. This is in the interest of the child, for the reasons mentioned above, so that unnecessary investigations and treatments are not embarked upon. A period of hospital admission also has other advantages such as identification of behavioural problems in the child and observation of parent-child interaction. During or after hospital admission, reported symptomatology may change as a result of the parent's contact with children who have other, more "impressive" symptomatology or diseases. For failure to thrive in infancy, which may occur as part of emotional abuse or neglect, a period of hospital admission to observe feeding behaviour and the ability to absorb adequately feeds, or gain weight is standard practice. Hospital admission or attendance may also be required for objective verification of reported allergic reactions by the use of double blind challenge tests (Warner and Haterway, 1984; Roesler *et al.*, 1994).

Detailed records should be made to document who collected/found specimens and from where. Laboratory analysis will help establish the nature of material reported to have come from a body orifice such as, stones or blood (DNA analysis). If further specimens are collected to verify abnormalities such as blood, these should ideally be collected by a nurse or other independent person, labelled and sent direct to the laboratory, ensuring the parent has no potential for intercepting the specimen's path (see example of fabricated sweat test, stool fat collection and sputum culture in a child *without* cystic fibrosis (Orenstein and Wassermann, 1986)). Similar methods should be used for collecting blood or urine for toxicology. If unknown, or complex substances are being administered, it can be helpful to contact a police forensic laboratory, which provides more extensive tests than most National Health Service (NHS) poisons laboratories (Rogers *et al.*, 1996). Salt poisoning requires a different analysis using simpler biochemical tests (Meadow, 1993).

If a child is admitted to hospital, detection of induced illness will be facilitated by keeping a record of all parent visits and activities, looking for temporal associations. Recurrent symptoms may warrant close observation with one-to-one nursing. This can be difficult to achieve as it requires ensuring that coffee and comfort breaks are covered by another nurse, and that no time is allowed with the nurse's back turned on the child in the mother's presence. Trips to the bathroom/toilet also need supervision. It may be possible to observe the child less intensively during a period of parental absence or exclusion. The latter is unlikely to be achieved voluntarily, but may be considered within a child protection plan when a high level of concern for serious harm exists.

For episodic life-threatening abuse, such as attempted suffocation or poisoning, where toxicology has proved negative, covert video surveillance may be helpful (Samuels *et al.*, 1992; Southall *et al.*, 1997; Rosen *et al.*,

1983; Boros *et al.*, 1995). This technique might also be useful in the detection of emotional abuse, where overt observations have been unhelpful in confirming suspicions of abuse. Alongside any of the above investigative routes, and particularly before undertaking covert video recordings, it is recommended that a multi-disciplinary planning meeting is held. This should preferably be in the form of a multi-agency strategy meeting chaired by social services. The use of such strategy meetings, without parents present, falls within the recommended guidance of the Department of Health (Social Services Inspectorate, 1994). Where parents are considered to be deceiving professionals, it is clear that working together may not be possible. To ensure adequate information is collected to protect the child, initial discussions need to be strictly confidential among those professionals who need to know.

The multi-agency strategy meeting provides a forum in which health, social services, education and police can share information about the family. It is not uncommon that the concerns relating to the medical issues in a child are only one piece of a jigsaw to which other agencies also provide information that gives concern. The presence of legal representation from social services at such a meeting is invaluable in providing a view as to whether there is sufficient information upon which to instigate child protection procedures, or whether further information needs to be collected. Participants in such a meeting need to be aware that if factitious illness is being considered, the parent may provide false information to other agencies and they too need to cross check information that they have obtained about the family with other agencies or colleagues in other parts of the country. Awareness that working together with parents may prove difficult ensures that the members of the strategy meeting obtain a high level of evidence before confrontation. This is why for episodic life-threatening abuse, strategy meetings have agreed to use covert video surveillance: for episodes which occur in hospital, this technique has a high detection rate for abuse (Southall *et al.*, 1997).

If a strategy meeting agrees that covert video surveillance is to be used, there are additional aspects of management that need to be agreed (see Table 2). It should be stressed that for such serious abuse, confrontation with the parent at this stage should be avoided, as this has been followed

Table 2. Decisions needed in planning meeting for covert video surveillance.

Management of patient prior to surveillance (e.g., one-to-one nursing supervision).
Training and briefing of observers (nurses, police officers) who will undertake surveillance.
Persons responsible for surveillance equipment and system for alerting ward staff.
Method of review of video tapes with suspected or actual harm.
Timing of and persons involved in review after specified duration (e.g., 72–120 h) of surveillance.
Subsequent management of child on detection of abuse.
Action to be taken if parent/carer attempts to remove child from ward, or if surveillance is negative.
Organisation of psychiatric assessment/support of parent/family.
Organisation of debriefing for staff.

by denial, discharge of the child, with subsequent return with a brain damaged or dead child (Waller, 1983; Meadow, 1990). Furthermore, denial without adequate information to support the existence of abuse is likely to be followed by the end of any therapeutic intervention by any agency.

Covert video recordings have been used since the early 1980s as an aid to the diagnosis of poisoning, attempted suffocation and emotional abuse (Samuels et al., 1992; Rosen et al., 1983; Epstein et al., 1987). Guidelines have been developed for the use of covert surveillance, and these help ensure that it is carried out safely and effectively (Southall and Samuels, 1996; Shabde and Craft, 1998). The use of such recordings provides legally admissable evidence (Williams and Bevan, 1988), and has been accepted in appropriately selected cases by the Royal College of Paediatrics and Child Health (British Paediatric Association Working Party, 1994), by Area Child Protection Committees, and by the Department of Health in the U.K. Moral, ethical and professional objections have been raised against the use of covert video surveillance and these are discussed elsewhere (Foreman and Farsides, 1993; Thomas, 1996; Evans, 1996; Morley, 1998), with replies (Southall and Samuels, 1993; 1995; Shinebourne, 1996). As in any potential child protection case, the welfare of the child is paramount (Bradley, 1998), and covert video surveillance may be the best mean to obtaining a diagnosis and protection of the child. Furthermore, the doctor has a professional duty to achieve where possible a diagnosis — failure to do so can result in further harm to the child, from both doctors and the abusing parent.

Covert video recordings can be made in an ordinary hospital cubicle, with 2–4 cameras hidden in the ceiling or walls of the cubicle (Samuels *et al.*, 1992; Southall *et al.*, 1997). In an adjacent office or room, video monitors and recorders permit continual observation of the well-being of the infant and allow the onset of any abusive behaviour to be documented and stopped. There need to be safeguards for the breakdown of any technical aspect of the video recording equipment. The observers of the recordings should be police officers or nursing staff, or preferably a combination of the two. They will have been informed in advance of the role of covert video surveillance and what particular abusive behaviour might be expected in the case they are observing. When harm, or potentially harmful actions are observed, they should alert ward staff to intervene in the cubicle, this taking no longer than 30 seconds from the onset of any serious episode. If there is doubt about the behaviour of the child, they can seek advice from the key paediatrician(s), social service and police staff who can review the tapes to assess whether sufficient evidence has been collected for child protection purposes (the aim is not primarily for a criminal level of evidence). When surveillance is used, it is important that there is a full briefing for the observers and all ward staff who may be involved in the intervention. The use of a debriefing meeting with the other agencies involved can also be helpful (Southall and Samuels, 1996).

In one report of 39 cases of children undergoing covert surveillance, child abuse was observed in 33 cases after a median duration of recording of 29 hours (range 15 minutes to 15 days) (Southall *et al.*, 1997). In 75% of cases, recordings were stopped by 60 hours. The mother (father in one case, grandmother in another), was observed to perform the abusive acts in a calm and calculated manner without any evidence that the child had in any way "provoked" the subsequent assault. Other observations from the video recordings showed either low levels of mother–child interaction, or very negative interactions which had not been overtly picked up by health professionals or social workers previously involved.

If serious abuse is observed, usual child protection procedures follow. The police will interview the abuser and a police or emergency protection order is obtained. Subsequently, a case conference will be convened where decisions about the future care of the child will be made. The abusing parent would usually have no unsupervised contact with the child and a careful assessment will be required of relatives who may be considered as future carers to the child.

The nature of evidence obtained from covert video recordings has meant that criminal convictions usually follow, thus ensuring that in the United Kingdom, the abusers are registered nationally as category one offenders. This is of value because the families involved in factitious illness have often moved from one area of the country to another making subsequent detection of abusive behaviour difficult.

The use of surveillance has been criticised because of the risk of further harm to the child (Morley, 1998). Even in hospital under surveillance, harm may occur (Klonnin, Samuels and Southall, 1996). The balance of risk for harm must be assessed, but for suspected and serious episodic abuse which remains unconfirmed, harm may be more likely to occur if the child is returned to the parent without detection. Furthermore, appropriate guidelines for using covert surveillance should ensure that any serious danger is minimised (Southall and Samuels, 1996).

Surveillance involves a betrayal of trust between paediatric staff and the child's parent. However, if the parent is deceiving health professionals, obtaining inappropriate hospital admission, investigations and treatment for their child and otherwise abusing the child, the use of surveillance may be justified as a quick, effective means for confirming the diagnosis (Shinebourne, 1996). Covert surveillance provides more definitive evidence, for example, than does a trial period of parental exclusion. There are of course many clinical situations where surveillance in hospital will not be appropriate. For example, if a young child shows developmental delay, behavioural and eating disorders then assessment after a trial period of alternative care may be a more appropriate means to achieving a diagnosis.

SUMMARY

There are various strategies that can be used to establish the validity of reported symptoms or cause of an illness. These range from a detailed exploration of the medical history through to sophisticated techniques such as the use of covert video surveillance. The decision as to which strategy to use depends in part on the frequency and severity of symptoms, an analysis of the likely harm involved, and an assessment of other issues that may affect parenting, such as abnormal illness behaviour and parental personality disorders. Such assessment cannot be undertaken by the paediatrician in isolation and it is important that full and confidential discussion between health professionals and the child protection team is central to the detection of this serious form of child abuse.

REFERENCES

Alexander, R., Smith, W., Stevenson, R. (1990). Serial Munchausen Syndrome by Proxy. *Pediatrics* **86**: 581–585.

Bools, C. N., Neal, B. A., Meadow, S. R. (1992). Co-morbidity associated with fabricated illness (Munchausen Syndrome by Proxy). *Arch. Dis. Child.* **67**: 77–79.

Bools, C. N., Neal, B. A., Meadow, R. (1994). Munchausen Syndrome by Proxy: A study of psychopathology. *Child Abuse Negl.* **18**: 773–788

Boros, S. J., Ophoven, J. P., Andersen, R., Brubaker, L. C. (1995). Munchausen Syndrome by Proxy: A profile for medical child abuse. *Australian Family Physician* **24**: 768–773.

Bradley, S. (1998). The child first and always. *Paediatric Nursing* **10**: 23–26.

British Paediatric Association Working Party. (1994). *Evaluation of Suspected Imposed Upper Airway Obstruction.* British Paediatric Association, London.

Bryk, M., Siegel, P. T. (1997). My mother caused my illness: The story of a survivor of Munchausen by Proxy Syndrome. *Pediatrics* **100**: 1–7.

Davis, P., McClure, R. J., Rolfe, K., Chessman, N., Pearson, S., Sibert, J. R., Meadow, R. (1998). Procedures, placement, and risks of further abuse after Munchausen Syndrome by Proxy, non-accidental poisoning and non-accidental suffocation. *Arch. Dis. Child.* **78**: 217–221

Donald, T., Jureidini, J. (1996). Munchausen Syndrome by Proxy. Child abuse in the medical system. *Arch. Pediatr. Adoles. Med.* **150**: 753–758.

Eminson, D. M., Postlethwaite, R. J. (1992). Factitious illness: Recognition and management. *Arch. Dis. Child.* **67**: 1510–1516.

Epstein, M. A., Markowitz, R. L., Gallo, D., Holmes, J. W., Gryboski, J. D. (1987). Munchausen Syndrome by Proxy: Considerations in diagnosis and confirmation by video surveillance. *Pediatrics* **80**: 220–224.

Evans, D. (1996). Covert video surveillance — a response to Professor Southall and Dr Samuels. *J. Med. Ethics* **22**: 29–32.

Feldman, M. D., Allen, D. B. (1996). "False-positive" factitious disorder by proxy. *South. Med. J.* **89**: 452–453.

Foreman, D. M., Farsides, C. (1993). Ethical use of covert videoing techniques in detecting Munchausen Syndrome by Proxy. *Br. Med. J.* **307**: 611–613.

Godding, V., Kruth, M. (1991). Compliance with treatment in asthma and Munchausen Syndrome by Proxy. *Arch. Dis. Child.* **66**: 956–960.

Jones, D. P. H., Lynch, M. A. (1998). Diagnosing and responding to serious child abuse. *Br. Med. J.* **317**: 484–485.

Jureidini, J. (1993). Obstetric factitious disorder and Munchausen Syndrome by Proxy. *J. Ner. Ment. Dis.* **181**: 137–139.

Klonnin, H., Samuels, M. P., Southall, D. P. (1996). Non-accidental fracture occurring in hospital. *Arch. Dis. Child.* **74**: 89–90.

Libow, G. A. (1995). Muchausen by Proxy victims in adulthood: A first look. *Child Abuse Negl.* **19**: 1131–1142.

Magnay, A. R., Debelle, G., Proops, D. W., Booth, I. W. (1994). Munchausen Syndrome by Proxy unmasked by nasal signs. *J. Laryngol. Otol.* **108**: 336–338.

Masterson, J., Dunworth, R., Williams, N. (1988). Extreme illness exaggeration in paediatric patients: A variant of Munchausen's by Proxy? *Amer. J. Ortho. Psychiat.* **58**: 188–195.

McClure, E. R. J., Davis, P. M., Meadow, S. R., Sibert, J. R. (1996). Epidemiology of Munchausen Syndrome by Proxy, non-accidental poisoning, and non-accidental suffocation. *Arch. Dis. Child.* **75**: 57–61.

McGuire, T. L., Feldman, K. W. (1989). Psychological morbidity of children subjected to Munchausen Syndrome by Proxy. *Pediatrics* **83**: 289–292.

Meadow, R. (1982). Munchausen Syndrome by Proxy. *Arch. Dis. Child.* **57**: 92–98.

Meadow, R. (1985). Management of Munchausen Syndrome by Proxy. *Arch. Dis. Child.* **600**: 385–393.

Meadow, R. (1993). Non-accidental salt poisoning. *Arch. Dis. Child.* **68**: 448–452.

Meadow, R. (1990). Suffocation, recurrent apnea, and sudden infant death. *J. Pediatr.* **117**: 351–357.

Morley, C. (1998). Concerns about using and interpreting covert video surveillance. *Br. Med. J.* **316**: 16–17.

Orenstein, D. M., Wassermann, A. L. (1986). Munchausen Syndrome by Proxy simulating cystic fibrosis. *Pediatrics* **78**: 621–624.

Poets, C. F., Samuels, M. P., Noyes, J. P., Hewertson, J., Hartmann, H., Holder, A., Southall, D. P. (1993). Home event recordings of oxygenation, breathing movements, and heart rate and rhythm in infants with recurrent life-threatening events. *Pediatrics* **123**: 693–701.

Roesler, T. A., Barry, P. C., Bock, S. A. (1994). Factitious food allergy and failure to thrive. *Arch. Pediat. Adolesc. Med.* **148**: 1150–1155.

Rogers, D., Tripp, J., Bentovim, A., Robinson, A., Berry, D., Goulding, R. (1976). Non-accidental poisoning: An extended syndrome of child abuse. *Br. Med. J.* **1**: 793–796.

Rosen, C. L., Frost, J. D., Bricker, T., Tarnow, J. D., Gillete, P. C., Dunlavy, S. (1983). Two siblings with recurrent cardiorespiratory arrest: Munchausen Syndrome by Proxy or child abuse? *Pediatrics* **71**: 715–720.

Rosenberg, D. A. (1987). Web of deceit: A literature review of Munchausen Syndrome by Proxy. *Child Abuse Negl.* **11**: 547–563.

Samuels, M. P., McClaughlin, W., Jacobson, R. R., Poets, C. F., Southall, D. P. (1992). Fourteen cases of imposed upper airway obstruction. *Arch. Dis. Child.* **67**: 162–170.

Shabde, N., Craft, A. W. (1998). Commentary: Covert video surveillance is acceptable — but only with a rigorous protocol. *Br. Med. J.* **316**: 17–18.

Shinebourne, E. A. (1996). Covert video surveillance and the principle of double effect: A response to criticism. *J. Med. Ethics* **22**: 26–28.

Siegel, P. T., Bryk, (1998). Munchausen by Proxy Syndrome. *Pediatrics* **101**: 951.

Social Services Inspectorate. (1994). *The Challenge of Partnership in Child Protection: Practice Guide*. Department of Health, HMSO.

Southall, D. P., Samuels, M. P. (1993). Ethical use of covert videoing for potentially life-threatening child abuse: A response to Drs Foreman and Farsides. *Br. Med. J.* **307**: 613–614.

Southall, D. P., Samuels, M. P. (1995). Some ethical issues surrounding covert video surveillance — a response. *J. Med. Ethics* **21**: 104–105.

Southall, D. P., Samuels, M. P. (1996). Guideline for the multi-agency management of patients suspected or at risk of suffering from life-threatening abuse resulting in cyanotic-apnoeic episodes. *J. Med. Ethics* **22**: 16–21.

Southall, D. P., Plunkett, M. C. B., Banks, M. W., Falcov, A. F., Samuels, M. P. (1997). Covert video recordings of life-threatening child abuse: Lessons for child protection. *Pediatrics* **100**: 735–760.

Thomas, T. (1996). Covert video surveillance — an assessment of the Staffordshire protocol. *J. Med. Ethics* **22**: 22–25.

Waller, D. A. (1983). Obstacles to the treatment of Munchausen by Proxy Syndrome. *J. Amer. Acad. Child Psych.* **22**: 80–85.

Warner, J. O., Hatherway, M. J. (1984). Allergic form of Meadow's Syndrome (Munchausen Syndrome by Proxy). *Arch. Dis. Child.* **59**: 151–156.

Williams, C., Bevan, V. T. (1988). The secret observation of children in hospital. *Lancet* **1**: 780–781.

CHAPTER 8

Assessment of Abusing Families

DAVID P. H. JONES, CAROLINE NEWBOLD

Park Hospital for Children, Oxford

Factitious Illness by Proxy (Munchausen Syndrome by Proxy) is a phenomenon, rather than a condition that afflicts an individual. The term Factitious Illness by Proxy (FIP) is used to describe situations where a parent or carer feigns an impression or produces a state of ill health in a child whom they are looking after. There are key elements of the phenomenon. Firstly, parental falsification or deceit concerning symptoms or signs of the child's ill health. Secondly, a triangular interaction between parent, child, and doctor, in which the doctor is misled by the parent, the child is harmed (either directly or indirectly), and some parental needs are met. Harm to the child occurs through one or more of the following ways: a) verbal fabrication of symptoms or signs, b) falsification of specimens, medical or nursing records, c) through inducing ill health (either through active means, or through withholding essential substances which lead to the child's ill health).

Conceptualised in this way, we can identify a number of different elements to this complex phenomenon (Jones and Bools, 1999); a) the harm caused to the child through fabrication, b) the impact on the child's development (including physical and/or emotional effects), and c) the mental state of the fabricator (including psychological condition, psychiatric diagnosis, as well as the consequences for parent/child interaction and attachment).

These aspects of FIP can have consequences in a number of areas, including child welfare, legal, and both adult and child mental health implications. In this chapter, we will set out our approach to assessment of children and families, based on the above conceptualisation of the phenomenon. We focus on those contributions which mental health services can make to the assessment. We identify two stages to assessment; the first is establishing whether a suspected situation is truly FIP or not — the diagnostic stage. The second is the subsequent evaluation of the psychological and social context, for case planning purposes. The first, diagnostic stage is usually undertaken by paediatricians, and much less frequently by social workers or police, or mental health services. The second stage includes the assessment of the fabricators' mental state and any emotional impact of FIP on the child and his or her siblings. We will contend that psychiatric services often have a role to play in the first stage, but are directly required during the second stage of assessment.

ESTABLISHING THE DIAGNOSIS OF FIP

There is an important role for the child psychiatric services to support nursing and medical staff while the diagnosis of FIP is being established. For paediatric teams to hold on to suspicion, while evaluating the possibility of FIP, can lead to considerable stress upon them. Paediatric nursing staff do not like being "detectives". They are naturally concerned lest the child is further harmed while the diagnosis is being confirmed. Psychiatric liaison with the paediatric team can be helpful while this difficult phase is being negotiated. The process of containing professional anxiety while suspicion is being evaluated is crucial if a firm diagnosis is to be made, because this provides the foundation for future case planning.

> For example, one mother was admitted to the paediatric ward with her baby of four weeks for full investigation of failure to thrive. All previous investigation had proved negative, and it appeared that, despite adequate food intake, the baby continued to lose weight alarmingly. The mother showed evidence of depression, and appeared to be relatively distant from her infant. The mother insisted on doing all feeds herself and her secrecy over the preparation of bottles raised suspicion among the nursing

staff that she might be tampering with the feeds. The psychiatric liaison enabled the nursing staff to be supported while they obtained samples of the mothers feeds from the refrigerator, and samples of the remainder of bottles which the infant did not wish to take. This enabled a firm diagnosis of deliberate dilution of feeds to be made (a form of FIP). Subsequent psychiatric assessment was thus feasible, and following intervention with mother and child together, successful reunification and child outcome resulted.

Situations which involve the possibility of covert video surveillance bring these issues into sharp relief. When this kind of assessment is contemplated, planning strategies which involve child psychiatric services as well as multidisciplinary case planning are essential.

Occasionally child and family psychiatric services are directly involved in the prediagnostic phase of FIP. An example is in the neuropsychiatric assessment of potential cases of Factitious Epilepsy by Proxy. In such cases, EEG monitoring, correlating EEG findings with video and clinical observations, and reported concerns of parents can establish the diagnosis.

For example, a mother who herself suffered from Munchausen Syndrome in the form of Factitious Epilepsy, had reported symptoms and signs of epilepsy in her seven-year-old child over several years. No one, besides the mother, had seen a seizure. All the child's examinations and EEGs were normal. However, due to the mother's persistence, antiepileptic medication had been prescribed. The child herself told her friends and teachers that she suffered from fits. During a two-week assessment admission ambulatory EEG monitoring was undertaken over four-day period, during which the mother reported several minor seizures and one major, tonic-clonic seizure. None of these were accompanied by EEG changes or clinical signs suggestive of a post-ictal state. A firm diagnosis of Factitious Epilepsy by Proxy was, in part, established through this assessment.

Once the paediatric diagnosis of FIP is established, child protection decisions will have to be made, in accordance with the procedures in the area. This will almost always involve the process of conveying the diagnosis to the parent. Sometimes the diagnosis is accepted, but more commonly righteous denial follows. If denial continues, the diagnosis is likely to be disputed and family justice proceedings will be contested. Expert opinions may be sought. There then may be considerable advantage in having a hearing on the medical facts alone, to sift through any difference of opinion concerning the diagnosis of FIP. Such a "split" hearing on the threshold criteria can provide a helpful basis for subsequent psychiatric assessment and therapeutic work with parents.

Sometimes psychiatric services are brought in during the assessment phase in order to provide psychiatric opinions about the fabricator, the child or other family members. More commonly, however, the contribution is consultative, working with paediatric nursing, medical and hospital social work colleagues, in the ways indicated above.

In summary, all paediatric services should have access to child and/or adult specialist psychiatric advice for severe abuse cases, including Factitious Illness by Proxy. In the past, paediatricians have found the involvement of psychiatric services in the assessment of cases of FIP to have been unhelpful sometimes. On occasions, it has appeared as though the psychiatric service has colluded with the fabricator's convincing denial, constituting a form of professional denial. We advocate psychiatric involvement from an early stage, working with paediatricians as closely as possible while assessing cases of severe abuse, especially FIP. There is major benefit for mental health professionals too, because they can then understand the dilemmas of their paediatric colleagues, the effect upon them and their teams, while also appreciating the severity of harm to the child in these cases. It is comparatively easy for mental health teams to "gaze avert" from the full nature of the abuse when the case comes to them, sanitised, and after any physical consequences have been treated. Furthermore, the basis of mutual trust between paediatric teams and psychiatric ones can be established through such liaison, providing an essential bedrock for psychosocial assessment, the second stage in the assessment process.

EVALUATION OF THE CHILD'S WELFARE AND PSYCHOLOGICAL STATUS

Following confirmation of a diagnosis of FIP, it is then the task of child protection agencies and mental health teams to plan for the future care and safety of the child who has been harmed. For consideration to be given to the option of family reunification in the aftermath of severe abuse we must make an assessment that change, focused on the child's welfare, is possible and feasible to achieve within a time frame which meets the developmental needs of the child. At the Park Hospital for Children in Oxford, we have been developing an assessment protocol to address the needs of these potentially dangerous families. The team's approach to assessment and treatment is grounded in an ecological/developmental perspective on severe parenting breakdown including child abuse and neglect (Jones, 1997) and incorporates concepts from the psychoanalytic, child development and attachment fields. As an overall goal, we seek a specific understanding of the origins of the FIP maltreatment in conjunction with a wider assessment of any other manifestations of parenting difficulty and/or different forms of abuse occurring within the family (Jones and Bools, 1999). Perhaps not surprisingly, it has become clear to us that a final outcome of factitious illness is reached by many different routes. For a person to resort to harming another in order to draw attention to their own distress, they will be influenced by a variety of factors related both to their individual personality and the way they form meaningful relationships with others. We may be able to identify a pattern of long-standing attachment difficulties and/or emotional abuse affecting the index child and frequently, although usually to a lesser extent, his siblings. In occasional cases, incidents of animal cruelty have also been discovered. The clinical picture as to the psychopathology of the perpetrator, the functioning of the family, the role of the non-abusing parent (usually father), the history and quality of the parent-child relationships, the nature and severity of the abuser, can be very varied from family to family and usually multifaceted.

The aim for psychiatric assessment is to determine firstly whether there is a focus for psychological treatment work and secondly to consider whether the patient's difficulties are matched by areas of personality strength which could enable them to engage effectively in treatment leading to significant change, in time for the child's developmental needs.

Jones and Bools (1999) have considered factors which contribute to the risk of recurrence or poor outcome in FIP cases. They present their analysis as a matrix of factors along six domains including child, parent and family factors. Our approach is to use this matrix for risk assessment and as a basis for setting criteria for change, when reunification is being considered.

Process of Assessment

The process of assessment is structured in such a way as to provide a number of points at which a decision can be made as to whether the family proceed to the next, more intense and extensive level or exit the programme because they are deemed to be unhelpable/untreatable.

The assessment process we have established aims to formulate as accurate and comprehensive a picture of the family as possible, in order to begin to consider the question of treatability. There is much to do in advance of an initial meeting with the family itself. A first crucial task will be to seek access to the medical records not only of the suspected perpetrator but of all family members in order to look for evidence of previous somatising behaviour and/or personality disturbance. In families with children older than the current index child, we may be able to detect a pattern of increasing harm with each subsequent child. This may only have come to professional attention at the point when severe abuse is discovered. Professional liaison with health and social service teams who have been involved in the detection and investigation process forms the other significant area of preparatory work in these high profile cases. The exact nature of all harm to the index child and his siblings must be clarified and understood. Inevitably, those who first treated a seriously sick or injured child or who had the task of securing the safety of the child at the point of initial crisis may feel sceptical about a psychiatric assessment regime aimed at determining the feasibility of family reunification. We attempt to address a range of professional views in the early stages of our assessment in order to establish an agreed series of concerns and in what way the situation will need to change (Jones, 1998). While we believe that child psychiatry has a significant role to play in planning for the future care of these children, their long-term safety will only be ensured as a result of effective multi-agency co-operation and effort. In order to avoid lengthy delay, the period prior to the legal statement of agreed findings of fact can be a time to gain an appreciation of general parenting difficulties and attachment relationships within the family. It is often possible to have an initial introduction to the family and to make a preliminary assessment of these areas without needing to focus on the abuse itself, the detail of which may remain incomplete at this stage.

Once the legal finding has been made, the assessment can extend its scope and consider the abuse as defined by the court. It should now be clear, on the balance of probabilities, that the harm suffered by the child was non-accidental. The most likely perpetrator may have been identified and the mechanism by which harm was done will have been made explicit. The task of the assessment at this stage is to elicit whether the abuse can be recognised and acknowledged within the family or whether a level of denial remains even after formal consideration of all the evidence. For those perpetrators who have organised their lives around the process of deception, it is now possible to counter this with an openness made feasible by the comprehensive legal hearing at which all parties have been professionally represented.

There will be some parents who continue to find it impossible to address the findings and even the non-abusing partner may be unable to concede the possibility of abuse, despite not being personally identified as culpable. Families who retain a high level of denial may have to be considered untreatable within a time-frame which addresses the child's need for permanency and security. Looking to the future, however, it is pertinent to make recommendations as to the help an individual might benefit from even if they are not likely to be a safe parent to the index child. There may be future children whose welfare must be considered at this early stage in the hope of avoiding repeat maltreatment.

For those parents who can acknowledge harming their child, it may still be an assessment challenge to help them recognise the full extent of the harm. For example, it can take time and careful work to help an abusing parent to understand that maltreatment has occurred within a context of severe attachment failure and breakdown of normal parenting capacity even if he/she can acknowledge specific incidents of harm. Similarly, enabling a parent to recognise less serious caretaking failures with a previous child may initially be unacceptable. However, even in the absence of a full acknowledgement in the initial stages, the family may be sufficiently motivated and engaged with the therapeutic team to be able to move into a more detailed assessment of the likely responsiveness to treatment in the longer term. At this point we often suggest a short (two-week) in-patient admission for the child and his closest family. In almost every case this will involve a disruption for the child from foster-care and at least a short-term family reunification although under highly supervised conditions. Hence, in order to propose this, we must be convinced that potential long-term safety and benefits derived from permanent reunification outweigh the temporary disruption.

The Family Unit's assessment procedure consists of a combination of informal observations, structured assessments and individual sessions with parents, undertaken by members of the multi-disciplinary team. As a cautionary measure for those of us working in a mental health setting, we have to take active steps to keep the reality of past maltreatment in mind, through written descriptions of the injury or harm caused to the child. By the time a child arrives on our unit their outward scars may have healed and the possibility of long-term damage may not yet have come to light.

All areas of the child's life and experience are assessed (Bryne and Jones, 1998; Jones, 1997; 1998) so that every aspect of potential future harm can be identified and its likelihood reduced. It is important to consider the possibility of harm of any kind not just that associated with factitious illness. Positive and negative features of parenting are recorded including observations of practical, psychological and emotional care. Assessments of everyday, ordinary activities which the parents and their children are engaged in, complement and inform sessions with individual family members.

It is our view that standardised psychological assessments should not be used in isolation as "tests" of parenting capacity. They are however useful in being able to challenge clinical assessments if results are discrepant.

In all observations of family interactions, particular attention is paid to the parent's sensitivity and responsiveness to the child's cues; the pattern and quality of attachment relationships; the parent's capacity for empathy with the child, and competency in all other aspects of parenting. Formal assessments will include the history of the parent-child relationship (which may extend to the time before conception) incorporating the parent's perception of the child and his conscious and unconscious meaning to her, as well as objective observable child factors including the child's developmental age, his state of mind, disposition and his capacity to engage with a care giver. In these ways, a comprehensive picture of the parent–child relationship is built up and changes closely monitored. This approach also facilitates a "child's eye view" (Jones, 1997) in which the team seeks to empathise with this particular child's experiences within his particular family. All our approaches are regularly co-ordinated in order to formulate an on going analysis of risk throughout the assessment and treatment phases.

Once the identified harm has been acknowledged and its context understood, we then expect to see an enhancement of parental sensitivity and competence during the inpatient period of treatment. Although this is moving now into the treatment phase of our work, we must constantly reassess progress towards change and the patient's ability to master and maintain more positively adaptive patterns of parenting. In this sense, assessment and treatment are inextricably linked.

The role of the non-abusing partner is crucial to this process of change. Their ability to identify future difficulties and seek appropriate help is of primary importance. To reach that stage, it will be necessary for the partner to not only acknowledge the fact of the abuse but also his/her role in the deception surrounding it. Their inability to protect the child within the context of FIP abuse needs to be considered and understood while some degree of therapeutic alliance established, aimed at sustaining change. Their feelings towards the abuser now will need careful recognition and assessment and decisions about the feasibility of an on going partnership must be addressed early on in the process. It would be very difficult, in these highly dangerous cases, to consider the return of a child to an abusing parent as sole carer, without the support and additional protection of another parent figure who has an understanding of past difficulties and who can be trusted to prioritise the needs of the child over and above those of his partner. Therefore, once a treatment phase has been embarked on, it is necessary to constantly reassess the feasibility of eventual safe reunification.

SUMMARY

Assessment continues throughout the life of a case of suspected FIP. Mental health services, both adult and child, have important contributions to make in all the different stages; at the beginning while the diagnosis is being established, and subsequently when the care and safety of the child is being assessed as to risk, and questions of family reunification are being considered. Psychological services need to be closely integrated with the work of other professionals and agencies at all stages. Child and family mental health services have a major contribution to make with these complex cases because of their focus on the child's development and overall welfare. All the signs are that cases involving FIP will need long-term follow-up, even if there has been successful family reunification, because while somatising behaviour can be successfully stopped, continuing problems with maternal mental health and the quality of parent/child interactions can persist and require further interaction (Jones and Bools, 1999). Nonetheless, for a minority of cases of FIP, family reunification is both feasible and a best option for the child and his or her siblings. The assessment challenge is to successfully identify those families with a relatively good prognosis as compared with the more persistently dangerous.

REFERENCES

Byrne, G., Jones, D. P. H. (1998). Inpatient assessment and treatment of severe breakdown in the parenting of infants. In Green, J. and Jacobs, B. (eds.). *The Inpatient Psychiatric Treatment of Children.* pp. 297–306 (Routledge, London).
Jones, D. P. H., Bools, C. N. (1999). Factitious Illness by Proxy. In David, T. (ed.). *Recent Advances in Paediatrics* 17, pp. 57–71 (Churchill Livingstone, Edinburgh).

Jones, D. P. H. (1997). Treatment of the child and the family where child abuse or neglect has occurred. In Helfer, R., Kempe, R. and Krugman, R. (eds.). *The Battered Child*, 5th edn., pp. 521–542 (University of Chicago Press, Chicago).

Jones, D. P. H. (1998). The effectiveness of intervention. In Adcock, M. and White, R. (eds.). *Significant Harm: Its Management and Outcome*, 2nd edn., pp. 91–119 (Significant Publications Ltd, Croydon).

CHAPTER 9

The Role of the Guardian Ad Litem

STEPHEN PIZZEY
Guardian Ad Litem and Social Work Consultant

The guardian ad litem is the independent person appointed by the court to represent and safeguard the interests of children in public law cases (also known as specified proceedings). Guardians ad litem are experienced social workers who have at least five years post-qualification experience. The guardian ad litem's duties are set out in the Children Act, 1989, the Family Proceedings Rules 1991, Part 4 (FPR 1991); and the Family Proceedings Courts (Children Act, 1989) Rules 1991 (FPC(CA1989) R 1991). The guardian ad litem must either be a member of a panel of guardians ad litem and reporting officers (administered either by single local authorities, consortia of local authorities or voluntary child care organisations under contract from a local authority); or the Official Solicitor. In practice, the Official Solicitor is rarely involved as guardian ad litem of the child in public law proceedings and in any event may only be appointed in these proceedings in the High Court.

COURT STRUCTURE AND PROCEDURE

Proceedings under the Children Act, 1989 are usually initiated in the Family Proceedings Court (Magistrates Courts). In the Family Proceedings Court, applications are heard by three lay magistrates advised by a court clerk or by a stipendiary magistrate. If there have been previous proceedings regarding the child in another tier of court, that is, County Court or High

Court, proceedings would usually be initiated at that court. In the County Court, applications are heard by a circuit judge.

Once the proceedings have been initiated they may be transferred from the Family Proceedings Courts to the County Court (in London this is the Principal Registry). The basis for such transfer would be to consolidate the application with other matters regarding the child already before the County Court, or urgency, exceptional complexity, gravity or importance. Cases may be transferred from the County Court level to the High Court if they are judged to be exceptional cases.

When considering the complexity of a particular case and therefore whether to transfer it to a higher court, consideration would be given to the following factors:

- the issues to be resolved regarding the likelihood of significant harm;
- differing interpretations of an explanation for serious injuries or medical problems;
- the level of risk to the child;
- the anticipated length of hearing;
- areas of disagreement between expert witnesses.

In practice, it is likely that cases of Munchausen Syndrome by Proxy would be transferred from the Family Proceedings Court to the County Court.

The length of time between an application being made and the final hearing of the case can vary. Because of the complexity of cases involving illness induction, it is likely that they will take in excess of six months. During the intervening period, the case is managed by the court via a series of directions appointments. In the Family Proceedings Courts, such directions appointments are heard by the court clerk, and in the County Court, by a district judge. At such appointments directions are made regarding the filing of evidence by the parties, appointment of experts, whether the child needs to attend court and so forth. A timetable will be organised in preparation for the final hearing, including the date of that hearing, and its length. Once all the documents, reports and statements have been filed with the court, a pre-trial review will be held before the court by the judge to clarify that the case is ready to be heard, the areas of law to be considered and any other matters that might need attention before the final hearing.

APPOINTMENT OF A GUARDIAN AD LITEM

Upon receipt of an application, the court is obliged to appoint a guardian ad litem unless it is satisfied that it is not necessary to do so in order to safeguard the child's interests (Children Act, 1989, Section 41(1)). The guardian ad litem should be appointed as soon as practicable after the commencement of any proceedings (FPR 1991, r 4.10(1)). Where a guardian ad litem has previously acted in respect of a child in previous proceedings, the court is required to consider appointing them to act again (FPR 1991, r 4.10(8)).

The proceedings in which a guardian ad litem can be appointed are set out in Section 41(6) of the Children Act, 1989. For the purposes of this chapter, the principal applications would be for a care or supervision order (Section 31), for the discharge or variation of a care order (Section 39(1), (2) and (4)), contact with a child who is the subject of a care order (Section 34), emergency protection order (Section 44), and any appeals (Section 41(6)(h)). The appointment of the guardian ad litem continues for the duration of the proceedings unless otherwise directed by the court or unless the appointment is terminated by the court (FPR 1991, r 4.10(9)).

POWERS AND DUTIES OF THE GUARDIAN AD LITEM

The guardian ad litem is under a duty to safeguard the interests of the child in the manner prescribed by Rules of Court (Section 41(2)(b) of the Children Act, 1989). Court rules (FPR 1991, r 4.11(1)) state that the guardian ad litem shall have regard to the principles set out in Section 1(2) of the Children Act, 1989 which states "in any proceedings in which any question with respect to the upbringing of the child arises, the court shall have regard to the general principle that any delay in determining the question is likely to prejudice the welfare of the child." The guardian ad litem is also required to have regard to the matters set out in Section 1(3)(a)–(f) of the Children Act, 1989 as if for the word "court" in that section there was substituted the words "guardian ad litem": (a) the ascertainable wishes and feelings of the child concerned (considered in the light of his age and understanding); (b) his physical, emotional and educational needs; (c) the likely effect on him of any change in his circumstances; (d) his age, sex, background and any characteristics of his which the court considers relevant; (e) any harm which he has suffered or is at risk of suffering; (f) how capable each of his parents, and any other person in relation to whom the court considers the question to be relevant, is of meeting his needs. The guardian ad litem is also required to advise on the options available to the court in respect of the child and the suitability of each such option including what order should be made in determining the application (FPR 1991, r 4.11(4)(e)).

The guardian ad litem is required to appoint a solicitor to represent the child unless a solicitor has already been appointed (FPR 1991, r 4.11(2)). The court may appoint a solicitor for the child where a guardian ad litem is not available in the first instance. The guardian ad litem is responsible for instructing the solicitor for the child (FPR 1991, r 4.11(2)(b)) unless the child is assessed by the solicitor to be able to give instructions on his own behalf (FPR 1991, r 4.12(1)(a)). Where a child has been assessed by the solicitor to be able to give instructions and there is a conflict between the instructions the child wishes to give and those that would be given by the guardian ad litem, the court may make a direction that the guardian ad litem should have separate legal representation.

The guardian ad litem is expected to advise the court (FPR 1991, r 4.11(4)):

- whether the child has sufficient understanding to give consent to a medical examination, psychiatric or any other assessment; the wishes of the child in respect to any matter relevant to the proceedings, including his attendance at court; which court the proceedings should be heard in and timing of the proceedings;
- the need for, and the relevant disciplines of, expert evidence; and
- any other matters concerning which the court seeks his advice or concerning which he considers the court should be informed.

The guardian ad litem, unless excused, is expected to attend all directions appointments and hearings and to provide advice to the court either orally or in writing (FPR 1991, r 4.11(5)). The guardian ad litem may be required to present interim reports on particular issues and a final report regarding all the matters before the court, specifically advising on the interests of the child (FPR 1991, r 4.11(7)). All parties to the proceedings have a right to question the guardian ad litem about any advice offered to the court either orally or in writing (FPR 1991, r 4.11(11)).

The guardian ad litem has additional duties to advise the court regarding possible parties to the proceedings who may in the interests of the child be joined to the proceedings (FPR 1991, r 4.11(6)). Where the child does not have a solicitor, the guardian ad litem is required to accept service of documents on behalf of the child, and where the child has sufficient understanding, to advise the child about the contents of such documents (FPR 1991, r 4.11(8)). Where a solicitor has been appointed, the solicitor accepts service of documents and where the child is instructing the solicitor, will advise the child of the contents of those documents. The guardian ad litem is also required to provide such other assistance to it as the court may require (FPR 1991, r 4.11(10)).

The guardian ad litem is required to investigate the matters before the court. Court rules (FPR 1991, r 4.11(9)) state:

"The guardian ad litem shall make such investigations as may be necessary for him to carry out his duties and shall, in particular —

(a) contact or seek to interview such persons as he thinks appropriate or as the court directs,
(b) if he inspects records of the kind referred to in Section 47 [principally local authority records regarding the child], bring to the attention of the court and such other persons as the court may direct all such records and documents which may, in his opinion, assist in the proper determination of the proceedings, and
(c) obtain such professional assistance as is available to him which he thinks appropriate or which court directs him to obtain."

The guardian ad litem may interview whoever he believes may be relevant to the investigation or such persons as the court directs provided the person concerned is willing to be interviewed.

The guardian ad litem has a right of access to local authority documents held regarding the child, is allowed to examine them and take copies of them (Section 42(1)2). The guardian ad litem does not have the right to examine hospital or doctors' records or records of other agencies held in respect of the child. Ordinarily the consent of someone with parental responsibility, that is, the parents or the local authority by virtue of an interim care order, would be required. Where this is not forthcoming, the guardian ad litem should raise this with the court at a directions appointment. The guardian ad litem does not have the right to inspect records held regarding parents or other family members. It is not unusual for the guardian ad litem to wish to see medical records of parents and their permission is required.

APPOINTMENT OF EXPERTS

The guardian ad litem must consider at an early stage whether the court requires any expert professional assistance. This may include paediatric examination, psychiatric assessment of the child and family functioning, developmental assessments of the child, psychiatric or psychological assessment of a parent or other significant adults. Such assessments may also be suggested to the court by other parties to the proceedings. Indeed, it is likely that the source of instructions for assessments of parents may well come from the parents' representatives rather than that of the guardian ad litem or local authority. Encouragement is given to parties to agree as far as possible the experts to be instructed and the questions to be asked of the expert. In general, the court would seek to avoid a duplication of experts from the same discipline.

No expert may be allowed to receive any of the documents in the proceedings without the leave of the court (FPR 1991, r 4.23). Leave of the court is also required for the child to be medically or psychiatrically examined or otherwise assessed for the purpose of the preparation of expert evidence for the use in the proceedings (FPR 1991, r 4.18(1)). The court's permission is not required for the examination of an adult but it is required for the release of documents. Guidance for experts reporting to the court in children's proceedings is provided in the Expert Witness Pack (1997). The guardian ad litem and other parties may consider whether a residential assessment or period of in-patient hospital assessment may be required. The relevance of and the funding of such assessments may be a matter of dispute between the parties. In certain circumstances courts have been known to direct local authorities under Section 38(6) to fund such assessments and for those assessments to take place during the course of the proceedings.

THE GUARDIAN AD LITEM'S REPORT AND RECOMMENDATION

Once the various experts who have been instructed have reported to the court and any Court directed assessments have been concluded, the local authority is given the opportunity to consider the reports and finalise its recommendations to the court and the plans for the child upon the making of an order. This plan is commonly known as the care plan. The parents and any other parties to the proceedings are given the opportunity to file further statements having considered the local authority's final statement and care plan. The guardian ad litem usually files his report after having received the aforementioned reports and statements. Guidance has been provided to guardians ad litem regarding the preparation of their reports (Pizzey and Davis, 1995; Munro and Forrester, 1995; Timms, 1991).

In the light of all the information provided the court, the guardian ad litem will be expected to examine closely the local authority's care plan and see if it meets the concerns raised in the proceedings and in the interests of the child whether it promotes their welfare and development. Guidance has been provided to local authorities in the preparation of care plans (Department of Health, 1991).

The guardian ad litem must consider which order or orders will best promote the child's welfare. In any application under the Children Act, the court "shall not make the order or any of the orders unless it considers that doing so would be better for the child than making no order at all" (Section 1(5)). The guardian ad litem must recommend the order or orders that would promote the welfare of the child. The court in a care order application may make the child the subject of a care order, conveying parental responsibility upon the local authority, a supervision order which initially lasts for one year, or no order at all. The court must also consider whether or not any contact orders should be made regarding the child. The local authority should state its contact proposals in its care plan. In general, the emphasis should be upon ensuring that the child is afforded reasonable contact with family members (Section 34(1)) insofar as it promotes and does not prejudice the child's welfare (Schedule 2, paragraph 15(1)).

When the court makes its final order or refuses the application, it must state any findings of fact and the reasons for its decision. If the final order is not in accordance with the recommendation of the guardian ad litem, he will consider with the child's solicitor whether or not to lodge an appeal. Appeals from the Family Proceedings Court are heard in the High Court. Appeals from the County Court are heard in the Court of Appeal.

REFERENCES

Pizzey, Davis, (1995). *A Guide to Guardians ad Litem in Public Law Proceedings under the Children Act, 1989.* HMSO, London.

Timms, J. (1991). *Manual of Practice Guidance for Guardians ad Litem and Reporting Officers.* HMSO, London.

Munro, Forrester, (1995). *The Guardian ad Litem.* Family Law (Jordan Publishing Ltd., Bristol).

Department of Health. (1991). *Children Act, 1989 Guidance and Regulations: Volume 3, Family Placements.* Paragraph 2.62, page 15. HMSO, London.

Expert Witness Group. (1997). *Expert Witness Pack.* Family Law (Jordan Publishing Ltd., Bristol).

The Family Proceedings Rules. (1991). HMSO, London.

The Family Proceedings Courts. (1991). (Children Act, 1989) Rules. HMSO, London.

CHAPTER 10

The Social Work Role in Munchausen Syndrome by Proxy

JENNY GRAY

Formerly Social Work Department,
Great Ormond Street Hospital for Children

Munchausen Syndrome by Proxy has been extensively documented in the medical and to a lesser extent, the psychiatric literature and is widely considered to be a health rather than a child protection issue. By comparison, the social work literature on this subject is sparse (Horwath and Lawson (eds.), 1995; Manthei *et al.*, 1988; Masterson and Wilson, 1987; Moeri *et al.*, 1996; Mercer and Perdue, 1993; Rees, 1987) although it is regarded as physical abuse in the English Government's inter-agency guidance on managing child protection, "Working Together to Safeguard Children" (Department of Health *et al.*, 1999). This chapter will focus on the social work role in the identification and management of Munchausen Syndrome by Proxy.

STATUTORY FRAMEWORK FOR SOCIAL WORK INTERVENTION

The Children Act 1989 provides the legal framework within which social workers employed by local authorities undertake their statutory duties in relation to children's welfare. (For the purposes of this book, key sections of the Children Act 1989 are summarised — see Appendix.)

THE CHILD PROTECTION PROCESS

When managing Munchausen Syndrome by Proxy cases, there is a growing body of knowledge for social work and other profesionals to draw on (Eminson and Postlethwaite, 1992; Gray *et al.*, 1995; Gray and Bentovim, 1996; Griffith, 1998; Horwath and Lawson (eds.), 1995; Jones *et al.*, 1986; Manthei *et al.*, 1988; Masterson and Wilson, 1987; Neale *et al.*, 1991; Rosenberg, 1987). In addition to following the local child protection procedures (Department of Health *et al.*, 1999; Department of Health *et al.*, 2000) the management of this type of child abuse case can be informed by research and clinical findings about the presenting signs and symptoms indicative of Munchausen Syndrome by Proxy; the common characteristics of the abuser and family; and the possible risks of significant harm to the child's life, health and development.

Identification of Cause for Concern

The focus of this chapter is on the identification of Munchausen Syndrome by Proxy in a paediatric context as this is normally where the evidence of child abuse becomes available. When all the medical tests are negative and/or members of the multi-disciplinary team become aware of information about the child and family which is congruent with the characteristics of Munchausen Syndrome by Proxy, the team including the social worker should consider the possibility of the signs and symptoms being caused by the induction of illness.

Once a suspicion of Munchausen Syndrome by Proxy has been raised, it is important for members of the multi-disciplinary team to discuss all the known information as in any other puzzling medical situation, to try and make sense of the child's symptoms. As part of the initial assessment, the team needs to plan what further medical investigations, staff observations and information about the child and family are required to understand the presenting symptoms and patterns of illness. During this information gathering period, it is vital that the results of all tests, investigations, and observations as well as verbal communications are accurately and fully recorded in the child's notes.

The local authority social worker has a statutory responsibility to bring together all the known information about the child and family (Department of Health *et al.*, 1999). This may involve the social worker seeking information from other local authorities which have information about the child, siblings, parents and extended family; the police to ascertain if the parents/adults in the household have any salient convictions or cautions; and any other agency which has information about the family, such as the health visiting, education and probation services and voluntary agencies. It is usual practice for the medical staff to contact other hospital consultants and GPs.

Strategy Discussion

If there is sufficient evidence of the child being harmed to consider making enquiries under section 47 of the Children Act, a strategy discussion involving key professionals should be convened by the Social Services Department. The purpose of the strategy discussion is to bring together all the information known at that time about the child, family and any agency involvement and consider whether to initiate a section 47 enquiry. If the evidence indicates there are grounds for doing so, the discussion then plans the enquiry allocating tasks to particular professionals. Although "Working Together to Safeguard Children" does not require a meeting, in my experience it is better to have one, as the complex issues raised in this type of abuse benefit from an exchange of information and discussion face-to-face. A meeting would normally be chaired by a social work manager from the local authority in which the child is residing at the time. Consideration of the welfare of the child must be of paramount importance (Children Act 1989) and therefore in cases of Munchausen Syndrome by Proxy, it is advised that parents be excluded from strategy discussions (Department of Health, 1995) in order to not place the children's lives at further risk of suffering significant harm, which in the most serious cases may lead to their death.

   If, at the strategy meeting, information is already available confirming that the child is being abused, it is essential to plan how best to protect the child whilst providing support to the abusing carer and to plan how and when the parents should be told of the child protection concerns. Future safety and interests of other children in the household should also be considered: the protection plans should include their need for protection.

Alternatively, it may be that more information is required and it is important to plan in detail how this information would be gathered, by whom and within what timescale. In order to ensure the child's protection, it is essential that all professionals involved with the child implement an agreed plan for carrying out the necessary investigations and observations. Further medical tests may be required or information sought from significant others who know the child and family. In some instances, it may be necessary for the child to be in a hospital setting where all the care is undertaken by the hospital staff.

The methods by which information is gathered will depend on the kinds of parental interference which could account for the symptoms or medical findings. Given the difficulties of collecting unequivocal medical evidence and managing Munchausen Syndrome by Proxy cases in ways that will ensure the child is protected, careful consideration must be given to the issues of separation from and contact with the main carer (Manthei *et al.*, 1988). This decision needs to be taken by the multi-disciplinary team and endorsed by the Social Services Department. In these types of cases the apparently most reasonable contact or communication arrangements can be used by the abuser to interfere with the child, specimens or equipment, and may be fraught with danger. If contact is being monitored for information gathering purposes, it is important to strike a balance between this process and the safety of the child, especially in situations where the child is possibly being smothered, poisoned or affected by a toxic substance. It may be necessary for the Social Services Department to apply for an Emergency Protection Order to ensure that the child is safe, pending a longer term child protection plan. As part of ensuring the child's safety, consideration should also be given to how the case will be managed if the abuse is confirmed. The Social Services Department should have a plan of action agreed, so that, if necessary, it can be put in place immediately after the identification of the abuse. This should include how and when to inform the parents (abusing parent and partner) of the evidence of abuse, the child of what is happening, how this information will be presented to them and who will undertake this task.

Section 47 Enquiries and Core Assessment

Where Munchausen Syndrome by Proxy is suspected, as in any other child abuse case, the Social Services Department has a duty to make enquiries about the child's welfare under section 47 of the Children Act, and these enquiries should be undertaken in accordance with the local authority's child protection procedures (Department of Health *et al.*, 1999; Department of Health *et al.*, 2000). Particularly in these types of abuse, the multi-disciplinary team needs to agree on a plan to:

- undertake any further medical and developmental tests, and observations on a child that are necessary to obtain objective evidence of the signs and symptoms;
- obtain a full medical, psychiatric and social history of all family members, with the information being validated at source;
- commence a core assessment which includes assessing family interactions, particularly those of the child with mother, other family members and professional staff;
- interview the child as appropriate to age and understanding regarding their perception of the symptoms and their causes;
- discuss with the parents the symptoms, child's history and professional concerns about not being able to identify through medical tests a satisfactory explanation for the alleged illness.

At this stage, the social work role is to commence a core assessment of the child, their relationships with family members, the family's functioning, attitude to the sick child, obtain a full social history and work with other members of the multi-disciplinary/multi-agency team. The Social Services Department has overall responsibility for ensuring that a section 47 enquiry is carried out, but all professionals should contribute according to the agreed strategy discussion plan.

The knowledge that in the absence of irrefutable medical evidence and the child being placed in a protective environment, telling the parents that Munchausen Syndrome by Proxy is suspected would put the child at even greater risk must be taken into account when considering the timing of this and who should be involved. Discussions with the parents must be undertaken at a point in time when the Social Services Department and medical plans are in place to ensure the safety and health of the child, other siblings, abusing parent and their partner. Each family member will have their own needs, which may not be compatible with one another, but which will require addressing.

One way of establishing a firm diagnosis of Munchausen Syndrome by Proxy is to separate the child from the suspected abuser for a specified period whilst continuing medical investigations and an assessment of the child. This can be undertaken on a voluntary basis with parental consent or as a consequence of the making of a court order. A decision to separate the child should be taken by the multi-disciplinary team, which includes a social worker. If this is part of the plan, careful thought needs to be given to how this matter is to be discussed with the parents in order that they have an understanding of the reasons behind such a decision and how the child will be given an explanation. At a minimum, the social worker and the consultant responsible for the child's care should be present when the parents are being spoken to, although I would recommend a senior member of the nursing staff to be present also as the ward nurses will have responsibility for the day-to-day management of the situation.

Child Protection Conference

If there is clear evidence that a child may continue to suffer or be at risk of suffering significant harm, then an initial child protection conference should be convened by social services according to the child protection procedures. If the abuse has been identified when the child is living in a local authority which is not that of their normal place of residence, the two social service departments need to agree on who will convene and chair the conference. It is essential that the social services department in which the child normally resides takes responsibility for the decisions made at the conference. The purpose of the conference is to decide whether the ACPC criterion is met for placing the child's name on the child protection register and if it is, to allocate the social worker who will undertake the key worker role; to agree an outline plan and the process by which a child protection plan is to be made; and what action will be taken immediately after the conference to ensure the child's safety. If the decision is not to place the child's name on the register, it is equally important to consider the child's needs and how best to offer support to the child and their family. McClure *et al.* (1996) in their national survey of Munchausen Syndrome by Proxy, non-accidental poisoning and suffocation cases in the United Kingdom and Eire during 1992–1994 found that paediatricians did not suggest convening a child protection conference until they considered they had concrete evidence of child abuse. The level of probability of the child having been abused based on medical evidence was a high as 90% which is higher than in normal diagnostic practice.

Prior to the child protection conference, the chair needs to decide whether it is in the child's interest for those with parental responsibility to attend all or part of the conference (Department of Health *et al.*, 1999; Department of Health, 1995). This will depend on the nature of the abuse, the dangers further abuse may present to the child's life and also on the extent to which each member of the professional team has been briefed about the facts of the abuse and been able to believe them. The protection of the child and the management of the case will be compromised by major splits between members of the multi-disciplinary team, and professionals in alliances with the parents. Hence the need for careful, early briefing of participants and access to a professional with specialist knowledge of this form of abuse.

Role of the Conference Chair

The conference chair will either be a Social Services Manager or an independent social worker appointed by the Department for this purpose. It is important that the conference chair ensures that some conference participants have specialist knowledge of Munchausen Syndrome by Proxy and before reaching a decision the following issues are considered by the participants:

- evidence of significant harm suffered by the child;
- an assessment of the nature and future risk of significant harm for the child drawing on research findings and clinical experience;

- past and future risk of significant harm to siblings;
- psychiatric histories of the abuser and family members, and the current status of mental health of the abusing carer;
- evidence of abuse including self-harm (Munchausen Syndrome by Proxy or Munchausen Syndrome in family members);
- verified historical details of illness, loss, bereavement, marital or parenting difficulties in the family;
- gains of having a sick child;
- degree of acknowledgement of the abuse by the abusing parent and other family members;
- denial or acceptance of the abuse by the professional network.

Outline Child Protection Plan

If the decision is to place the child's name on the child protection register, a child protection plan will need to be constructed based on the findings of the core assessment. An outline plan will need to be in place to take effect from the time the conference ends to ensure the child's safety. The discussions at the conference should draw on research and practice-based knowledge about Munchausen Syndrome by Proxy and specifically address the following issues:

- Will the child be protected if placed with the abusing parent? How would this be monitored effectively?
- Will the child be protected if placed with family members, and particularly those related to the abusing parent?
- What type of contact should the child have with the abusing parent, given the way in which the child is abused, for example, smothered, poisoned, symptoms fabricated, food actively withheld?
- If the child is not to return home, what will be the statutory basis on which the child will be looked after and who will brief the new carers on the nature of illness induction, contact arrangements and possible ways in which the abuser could continue to induce illness?
- Who will brief those not present at the conference on the evidence of abuse ensuring they understand the future risks to the child, rationale

for decisions and if necessary, their future role (statutory and therapeutic) with the child and family?

- What explanation of the conference decisions will be given to the child, parents and siblings, in a manner which is therapeutically helpful?

Core Assessment

When a section 47 enquiry is initiated, the Social Services Department has lead responsibility for undertaking a core assessment of the child and their family and ensuring that other professionals contribute according to the agreed plan. If a child protection conference has been convened and the child's name is placed on a child protection register the core assessment continues. It should be completed within a maximum of 35 working days (Department of Health *et al.*, 2000). Ideally, the core assessment should include an assessment of the abusing parent's mental health and the functioning of the family system by a child and family psychiatrist, preferably one with expertise in Munchausen Syndrome by Proxy. If care proceedings have been initiated, this assessment will inform the Social Services Department's Care plan being constructed for the Court. As part of the therapeutic process, the professionals involved need to develop an understanding of the way in which the pattern of abusive behaviour has evolved and its function within each family system to decide how best to protect the child and to manage this type of child abuse situation (Gray and Bentovim, 1996; Griffith, 1988; Manthei *et al.*, 1988). This understanding will be derived from an analysis of all the known information about the child's medical history and characteristics as well as the medical, psychiatric and social history of all family members. The gain for most perpetrators of Munchausen Syndrome by Proxy seems to be the attention, and proxy nurturing they receive from health professionals as the carer of a "sick" child, often over long periods. They are said to experience a hospital or health care environment as supportive and report feeling unusually important and respected in that milieu. For some, respect and status in their community may emanate from being the parent of a child with an obscure or medically baffling illness. The family may have become the focus for much fund raising activity and publicity. Thus the community system may serve to reinforce the benefits received by the family through having a sick child.

Child Protection Plan

If the child's name is placed on the child protection register, the Social Services Department, through the key worker, has overall responsibility for ensuring that a plan is constructed and carried out. A number of different professionals will have responsibility for carrying out aspects of the plan. The plan will need to be reviewed and revised as the child and family's circumstances change, initially three months after the initial child protection conference and thereafter at least every six months (Department of Health *et al.*, 1999).

- The plan needs to address the immediate, short and long term needs of the child and each family member, taking account of the factors which are associated with a good outcome for the child (Gray *et al.*, 1995). Intensive therapeutic input will be required in the period after identification, and over time this should be able to be reduced in intensity and the child's life normalised.
- The plan needs to have realistic goals, and appropriate timescales, taking account of the needs and age of the child. However, the timescales within which the abusing parent may make therapeutic progress may be incompatible with the child's long-term needs for family stability.
- The plan needs to be based on a multi-disciplinary in-depth assessment of the needs of the child and all family members and be informed by knowledge of the outcomes of therapeutic help or non-intervention.
- The plan should set out the specific work that needs to be undertaken by professionals and family members in order to ensure that the child's needs are met. It may include individual work with the child (including in-patient treatment); individual work with the mother; therapeutic help with parenting, relationship and family issues.
- The plan should set out what therapeutic help will be offered to the abusing parent. If possible a child and family psychiatrist with experience of Munchausen Syndrome by Proxy should be involved.

- If other children remain in the care of the parent responsible for the abuse, a system appropriate to the type of abuse should be set up to monitor their safety and ensure that they are not also being abused.
- If a child is placed out of the family home, and it is subsequently considered to be safe to try to reunite the child with their family, this process needs to be carefully monitored. It is important to use objective measures appropriate to each child to monitor their outcomes.

Those who have identified the abuse need to work closely with other members of the inter-agency, inter-professional network to help them understand how the maltreatment was carried out and the harm it caused the child. In some situations, professionals may enter into a collusive relationship with the parents, in particular the mother. This impairs their ability to intervene and ensure the child is protected when living within their family context.

Outcomes for Children

Successful reunification involving a safe return home of the child will require evidence of significant change in the abusing parent and within the family system as a whole. The allocated social worker needs to collate the information available for use when deciding whether this is possible. There is overwhelming evidence (Bools et al., 1992; Gray et al., 1995; Jones et al., 1986; Meadow, 1993; Neale et al., 1991) that when a child is placed in a life threatening situation it is extremely difficult to achieve, particularly within a timescale that renders a permanent return to the original nuclear family realistic and indeed such a change may be impossible. However, there are examples of planned therapeutic work having a good outcome for the child which includes returning home to the care of the abusing parent (Black and Hollis, 1996; Coombe, 1995; Nicol and Eccles, 1985; Gray et al., 1995; Gray and Bentovim, 1996; Sanders, 1996). These can be drawn on when considering how to intervene in order to bring about the required change.

In a study of 41 children where Munchausen Syndrome by Proxy had been identified and managed by the same hospital, there were four deaths, two of which occurred as a direct result of the child abuse (Gray et al.,

1995). The findings of this review suggested that the way in which the cases are managed relates directly to the outcomes for the children. There was evidence of a good outcome for 16 (39%) of the surviving children in situations where cases were managed within a child protection framework, therapeutic interventions were focused on the protection of the child, an in-depth assessment was undertaken of the family's functioning and its ability to change and protect the child, and clear decisions were made about whether the child was able to live with both parents, the non-abusing parent or should be placed in an alternative family context.

Successful outcomes for children requires professionals to maintain a clear focus on the child's safety and welfare at all stages in the child protection process.

APPENDIX — SUMMARY OF RELEVANT SECTIONS OF THE CHILDREN ACT, 1989

Section 17: Children in Need

Section 17 addresses the duty of the local authority to provide services for "children in need, their families and others". Section 17(1) states

"it is the general duty of every local authority…

(a) to safeguard and promote the welfare of children within their area who are in need; and
(b) so far as is consistent with that duty, to promote the upbringing of such children by their families, by providing a range and level of services appropriate to those children's needs."

Section 17(10) states that for the purposes of this part of the Act a child should be taken to be in need if —

(a) "he is unlikely to achieve or maintain, or to have the opportunity of achieving or maintaining, a reasonable standard of health or development without the provision for him services by a local authority under this part;

(b) his health or development is likely to be significantly impaired, or further impaired, without the provision for him of such services; or

(c) he is disabled,

and 'family', in relation to such a child, includes any person who has parental responsibility for the child and any other person with whom he has been living."

Sub-section 11 also goes on to say that for the purposes of this part of the Act:

"a child is disabled if he is blind, deaf or dumb, or suffers from any mental disorder of any kind or is substantially or permanently handicapped by illness, injury or congenital deformity or such other disability as may be prescribed; and in this Part —

'development' means physical, intellectual, emotional, social or behavioural development; and

'health' means physical or mental health."

Services provided by the local authority to a family are generally referred to as Section 17 services. They are provided as part of an agreement with the family in order to assist in meeting the needs of each child who is a family member. In situations where Munchausen Syndrome by Proxy is identified, children may have been in receipt of services from a local authority but there had been no prior suspicion of illness having been induced by a carer or symptoms fabricated. They may have had a social worker allocated under S17 of the Children Act. There will also be a group of cases, where the social worker has begun to doubt the veracity of the carer's claims but there is no clear evidence of abuse. In other family situations, perhaps the majority, the child and family will not be known to social services or past involvement may have been minimal or some time ago.

Section 47 Enquiries

The local authority's duty to investigate is commonly referred to as section 47 enquiries and are set out in Section 47(1) which states:

"Where a local authority —

(a) are informed that a child who lives, or is found, in their area —

  (i) is the subject of an emergency protection order; or
  (ii) is in police protection; or

(b) have reasonable cause to suspect that a child who lives, or is found, in the area is suffering, or is likely to suffer significant harm,

the authority shall make, or cause to be made, such enquiries as they consider necessary to enable them to decide whether they should take any action to safeguard or promote the child's welfare."

Under section 47, the local authority has a responsibility to make enquiries when they are informed about a child who lives or is found in their area. This means that the local authority in which the child is living or "staying" at the time that the abuse is identified has responsibility for ensuring the section 47 enquiry is carried out. In situations, as is often the case with Munchausen Syndrome by Proxy where the abuse is identified in a specialist hospital in one local authority and the child ordinarily resides in another local authority, it is the responsibility of the local authority in which the hospital is situated to initiate the section 47 enquiry. Good practice would suggest that the two local authorities (of the hospital and of the children's normal place of residence) agree a *modus operandi* in which one has clear statutory responsibility for the section 47 and an agreement is reached on who from which local authority will undertake it and any further statutory involvement. This will also mean agreeing how to work to two ACPC child protection procedures which may differ in their detail.

Working Together to Safeguard Children

The process from identification of a child protection concern through to, if appropriate, conducting section 47 enquiries, holding child protection conferences, placing the child's name on a child protection register, reviewing this decision and deciding to remove the child's name is undertaken according to the government guidance set out in "Working Together to Safeguard

Children". This guidance was issued under Section 7 of The Local Authorities Social Services Act, 1970 which requires "local authorities and their social services functions to act under the general guidance of the state. As such, this document does not have the full force of statute, but should be complied with unless local circumstances indicate exceptional reasons which justify a variation."

Part V of the Children Act 1989

Part V of the Children Act 1989 deals with the protection of children. In situations where immediate action is required to protect a child, an emergency protection order can be sought under section 44 or the police may take action under section 46 to ensure a child is safe. In practice, it is the local authority which applies for an emergency protection order when:

(a) "there is reasonable cause to believe that the child is likely to suffer significant harm if —

  (i) he is not removed to accommodation provided by or on behalf of the applicant; or
  (ii) he does not remain in the place in which he is then being accommodated." (Section 44(1)).

If the order is granted, the child can either be moved to a safe place, for example a foster home, or remain in a safe place, for example a hospital. Making the order also confers on the local authority parental responsibility for the child but does not remove it from anyone who already had it, for example, the mother. An emergency protection order lasts for a maximum of eight days but can be extended for a further seven days if necessary (Section 45). A child can only be kept in police protection for 72 hours, during which time decisions need to be made by the Social Services Department regarding the child's future — to remain at home, be accommodated by the local authority, or apply for an emergency protection order under section 44.

Under section 43, the local authority can apply for an assessment order which can last for a maximum of seven days from the date specified on the order. This Section could be used where:

(a) the applicant has reasonable cause to suspect that the child is suffering or likely to suffer significant harm;
(b) an assessment of the state of the child's health or development or of the way in which he has been treated, is required to enable the applicant to determine whether or not the child is suffering, or is likely to suffer, significant harm; and
(c) it is unlikely that such an assessment will be made, or be satisfactory, in the absence of an order under this section. (Section 43(1)).

The original intention was that the assessment order could be used in situations where there was grave concern about the child's welfare but insufficient evidence available due to the parents' refusal to allow an assessment of the child to be carried out, leading to lack of clarity about whether or not the child was suffering or likely to suffer significant harm. In practice, this section of the Children Act has been rarely used since the implementation of the Act in October 1991. It would seem that information is obtained either by agreement with the parents or where the local authority has assumed parental responsibility for the child following the making of a statutory order such as an emergency protection or an interim care order.

When the child has been made the subject of an emergency protection order or is in police protection, the local authority has a duty to make enquiries about his welfare (under section 47) and decide what action to take in order to "safeguard or promote the child's welfare". The local authority may apply for either a care or a supervision order with respect to a child who is under 17 years (or 16 if the child is married) subject to the Court being satisfied:

(a) that the child concerned is suffering, or likely to suffer, a significant harm; and
(b) that the harm, or likelihood of harm, is attributable to —

   (i) the care given to the child or likely to be given to him if the order is not made, not being what it would be reasonable to expect a parent to give him; or
   (ii) the child is beyond parental control. (Section 31(2)).

The making of this order confers parental responsibility on the local authority but does not remove parental responsibility from those who already have it. Under section 34(1)(a), where a child is in the care of the local authority, it "shall allow the child reasonable contact with parents subject to the provision of the section". In Munchausen Syndrome by Proxy cases, the nature and frequency of a child's contact with the abusing parent is a major issue, as the seemingly most innocent forms of contact, even when closely supervised, can be dangerous to the child. The usual pattern would be for a number of interim care orders to be made under Section 38(1) until such time as the court has sufficient information on which to make a final decision. Where the court makes an interim order, it may give directions as it considers appropriate "with regard to the medical or psychiatric examination or other assessment of the child" (Section 38(6)). In all decisions made by the court, the welfare of the child is of paramount consideration (Section 1). The Court will have particular regard to what is known as the welfare checklist —

(a) the ascertainable wishes and feelings of the child concerned (considered in the light of his age and understanding);
(b) his physical, emotional and educational needs;
(c) the likely effect on him of any change in his circumstances;
(d) his age, sex, background and any characteristics of his which the court considers relevant;
(e) any harm which he has suffered or is at risk of suffering;
(f) how capable each of his parents or any other person in relation to whom the court considers the question to be relevant, is of meeting his needs;
(g) the range of powers available to the court under this Act and the proceedings in question.

In preparing their reports for the court, both the social worker and the guardian ad litem will need to address these areas. The local authority decides its care plan following careful consideration of all the available information and having made judgements about what action will be in the child's best interests. The use of all the available research and clinical evidence is crucial to this decision making process.

If the abuse has been identified, it is the responsibility of the local authority to provide whatever social care services have been agreed under the child protection plan following the child's name being placed on the child protection register, and to exercise its parental responsibility to the child if he is the subject of an emergency protection order or an interim care order. The court can make the child the subject of a supervision order (Section 35(1)) which means it is a duty of the person supervising the order to "advise, assist and befriend the supervised child", but in practice these orders are rarely made. In Munchausen Syndrome by Proxy cases, it can be helpful to substitute a supervision order for a care order if the intention is to continue to offer support to the child and their family after a more intensive period of intervention when the child was the subject of a care order.

REFERENCES

Black, D., Hollis, P. (1996). Psychiatric treatment of factitious illness in an infant (Munchausen by Proxy Syndrome). *Clin. Child Psychol. Psychiatry* **1**: 89–98.

Bools, C. W., Neale, B. A., Meadow, S. R. (1992). Co-morbidity associated with fabricated illness (Munchausen Syndrome by Proxy). *Arch. Dis. Child.* **67**: 77–79.

Children Act 1989, (HMSO, London).

Coombe, P. (1995). The in-patient psychotherapy of a mother and child at the Cassel Hospital: A case of Munchausen's Syndrome by Proxy. *Br. J. Psychother.* **12**: 195–207.

Department of Health. (1995). *The Challenge of Partnership in Child Protection: Practice Guide.* HMSO, London.

Department of Health, *et al.* (1999). *Working Together to Safeguard Children. A Guide to Inter-agency Working to Safeguard and Promote the Welfare of Children.* The Stationery Office, London.

Department of Health, *et al.* (2000). *Framework for the Assessment of Children in Need and their Families.* The Stationery Office, London.

Eminson, D., Postlethwaite, R. (1992). Factitious management: Recognition and management. *Arch. Dis. Child.* **67**: 1510–1516.

Gray, J., Bentovim, A. (1996). Illness Induction Syndrome: Paper 1 — A series of 41 children from 37 families identified at the Great Ormond Street Hospital for Children NHS Trust. *Child Abuse and Negl.* **20**: 655–673.

Gray, J., Bentovim, A., Milla, P. (1995). *The Treatment of Children and Their Families where Induced Illness has been Identified*, eds. Horwath and Lawson (National Children's Bureau, London) 149–162.

Griffith, J. (1988). The family systems of Munchausen Syndrome by Proxy. *Family Process* **27**: 423–437.

Horwath, J., Lawson, eds., *Trust Betrayed, Munchausen Syndrome by Proxy, Interagency Child Protection and Partnership with Families*, (National Children's Bureau London, 1995).

Jones, J. G., *et al.* (1986). Munchausen Syndrome by Proxy. *Child Abuse and Negl.* **10**: 33–40.

Manthei, D. J., *et al.* (1988). Munchausen Syndrome by Proxy: Covert child abuse *J. Fam. Viol.* **3**: 131–140.

Masterson, J., Wilson, J. (1987). Factitious illness in children: The social worker's role in the identification and management. *Social Work in Health Care* **12**: 21–31.

McClure, R. J., Davis, P. M., Meadow, S. R., Sibert, J. R. (1996). Epidemiology of Munchausen Syndrome by Proxy, non-accidental poisoning, and non-accidental suffocation. *Arch. Dis. Child.* **75**: 57–61.

Mercer, S. O., Perdue, J. D. (1993). Munchausen Syndrome by Proxy: Social work's role. *Social Work* **38**: 74–81.

Moeri, V., Gray, J., Rawlings, D. (1996). The identification and management of Illness Induction Syndrome. *Practice* **8**: 27–42.

Neale, B., Bools, C., Meadow, R. (1991). Problems in the assessment and management of Munchausen Syndrome by Proxy abuse. *Children and Society* **5**: 324–333.

Nicol, A. R., Eccles, M. (1985). Psychotherapy for Munchausen Syndrome by Proxy. *Arch. Dis. Child.* **60**: 344–348.

Rees, S. V. (1987). Munchausen Syndrome by Proxy: Another form of child abuse. *Practice* **3**: 267–283.

Rogers, D., *et al.* (1976). Non-accidental poisoning: an extended syndrome of abuse. *Br. Med. J.* **1**: 793–796.

Rosenberg, D. (1987). Web of deceit: A literature review of Munchausen Syndrome by Proxy. *Child Abuse and Negl.* **11**: 547–563.

Sanders, M. J. (1996). Narrative family treatment of Munchausen Syndrome by Proxy: A successful case. *Families, Systems and Health* **14**: 315–329.

CHAPTER 11

Munchausen's Syndrome by Proxy — The Legal Perspective

DEBBIE TAYLOR
Barrister at Law of Lincoln's Inn, London

MICHAEL NICHOLLS
Barrister at Law of Middle Temple, London

INTRODUCTION

A suggestion that a child has been the victim of Munchausen Syndrome by Proxy (MSBP) or "Factitious Disorder by Proxy" as it is sometimes called now, is so serious that it will almost without exception cause the local authority within whose area the child usually lives or happens to be, for instance for medical treatment, to consider instituting protection proceedings under the Children Act, 1989 with a view to taking the child into care. If an allegation or suspicion that a child has been the victim of MSBP arises within what are known as "private law" proceedings between the child's parents or other members of the family about the child's upbringing, the court will almost certainly want to involve the local authority, because if the allegation is true, the child might have to be taken into care. If the case is in the County Court, the judge will give very serious consideration to transferring it to the High Court, and appointing the Official Solicitor to act for the child.

One of the reasons that an allegation of MSBP is taken so seriously is not that it necessarily involves unusually cruel treatment of a child, although the mortality rate is quite high and there is a serious danger to siblings, but that it is so difficult to prove. However, MSBP covers a wide range of behaviour from the excessively anxious parent exaggerating minor symptoms and encouraging a feeling of guilt in a child who otherwise feels well, through neglect or cruelty coupled with denial, to administering poison or caustic substances and interfering with medication. The term MSBP is "now usually restricted to the more extreme end of the spectrum" (Kelly and Loader, 1997), and care must be taken not to allow a "label" or diagnosis to influence the way in which the case is conducted. If the case is really one which used to be called "cruelty", it should be dealt with accordingly. Another difficulty is that perpetrators may be very plausible, co-operating fully with the medical staff, and often becoming involved in the life of the hospital and the ward. Not all show the warning signs of self-harm, drug or alcohol abuse, frequent changes of GP and multiple admissions to different hospitals.

As the perpetrator is often the child's main carer, it is especially difficult to determine the extent to which the perpetrator's partner, usually the father, has colluded with the perpetrator and failed to protect the child. If the medical staff have taken so long to find out what was going on, how could the father have known? Deciding whether it is safe to leave the child with one of its parents, or whether removal from its family is the only choice are extremely difficult and onerous decisions, as are the decisions about contact between the child and both its parents.

THE DIFFICULTIES OF PROOF

The primary problem that faces the courts is proving that the child has been the victim of the syndrome. Once the problem has been identified, sophisticated expert evidence is inevitably required before a final decision is made by the court about what to do. However at the outset, the problem is one of evidence. Proceedings about the care and welfare of children are family proceedings. The rules of evidence in family proceedings are quite generous so that, for example, hearsay evidence is admissible and the proceedings are generally regarded as being more inquisitorial than adversarial. No-one is supposed to be "on trial", the object being to do what is best for the child. However, it is unrealistic to expect parents who are accused of causing their child so much damage to regard themselves as anything other than being on trial, especially as criminal charges may well also be brought.

When Parliament comprehensively reformed the law relating to the protection of children in the Children Act, 1989, it did away with the many different ways in which a child could previously have been taken into care and put in their place a single route into care by proof of significant harm. In addition, the usual rules about legal proceeding apply, in that the party who makes an allegation must prove it to the evidential standard applicable to the proceedings — what is known as carrying the legal and evidential burden.

Accordingly, when a local authority makes an application for a care order, it must prove that the child is suffering or likely to suffer significant harm which is attributable to the care being given to him, or likely to be given to him if the order is not made, not being what it would be reasonable to expect a parent to give him, or because he is beyond parental control (Children Act, 1989, Section 31(2)). Further, where the question of whether harm suffered by a child is "significant" turns on the child's health or development, his health or development has to be compared with that which could reasonably be expected of a similar child (Children Act, 1989, Section 31(10)). Having set significant harm as being the criteria for the intervention of the state in family life, Parliament did not go on to fix the standard of proof, but by inference left it at the civil standard, that is, the balance of probabilities. Only recently has the House of Lords in the case of *Re H and R* (*Child Sexual Abuse: Standard of Proof*) [1996] 1 FLR 80 had to reiterate that mere suspicion is not enough to justify making a care order, and that significant harm had to be proved.

PROCEDURE AND EXPERT EVIDENCE

Cases involving allegations of MSBP have given rise to a number of reported decisions in the field of family law, one of which, *Re P* (*Emergency Protection Order*) [1996] 1 FLR 482, might be described as a classic case, and illustrates both the legal process and the evidential difficulties. The child, M, was born in October 1994, and on 7 and 8 December 1994, there were two episodes when he nearly died. The paediatrician who attended to him suspected that his mother had tried to suffocate him. The local authority obtained an emergency protection order, which had to be renewed on 29 December 1994. The justices in the family proceedings court refused to extend the order. There were then extensive and prolonged investigations carried out by a number of experienced paediatricians, including consultants instructed on behalf of the parents, culminating in a brain scan. Those investigations confirmed the original view that there had been no medical cause for what had happened, and the medical experts arrived at a consensus that, there being no medical cause for what happened, the overwhelming probability was that the child's mother smothered him in some way in some quick moment of time which no one could identify for sure. In addition, the mother has given accounts of what happened which contained inconsistencies and she had said things which were patently and obviously untrue as, for example, by asserting to the doctors that she was qualified as a nurse.

The mother was diagnosed as having MSBP, but the judge said that "for the court, the question is not to make a particular diagnosis, but to identify what happened to the child concerned and what should happen in the future." The parents withdrew their objection to a care order being made, and the local authority took a bold course, continuing to "hope that [the child] can make his home where he truly belongs, that is to say, at home with his family; that the mother in particular will receive help to overcome the problem that she has. Illness, disability and incapacity take many forms. This is not a mother who anyone should think should be blamed for what happened. She is a loving, caring and committed mother. She deserves the sympathy of all of us and she deserves to receive whatever help can be provided by appropriate professionals."

The case highlights some of the legal and practical difficulties which arise. As they approached the end of their investigations, the doctors wanted to eliminate the possibility that the child's difficulties with breathing on the two major occasions were caused by spasms resulting from some specific form of epilepsy. In order to eliminate that possible cause, it was necessary for an appropriately experienced doctor to examine a scan of part of his brain. A dispute then arose about funding the modest cost of that examination, which was only resolved by the judge indicating that it would be a proper legal aid disbursement. There was also the problem that there seemed to be no way in which the local authority could challenge the justice's refusal, probably as a result of misunderstanding the expert medical evidence, to extend the Emergency Protection Order.

As to evidence, the judge said that "in these cases the court has to be satisfied of what is alleged on the balance of probabilities, but the cogency of the evidence necessary to tip the balance in favour of the allegation must be consistent with the gravity of the allegation made. There can surely be no graver an allegation than is made here. However, on the basis of the medical evidence, but also coupling with that the other evidence in the case, I express myself as being sure that the mother was responsible for what happened to M. There is no other basis for the making of the care order that is sought other than these events. It is important for the future that I should record plainly my finding in the matter. M suffered significant harm in the care of his mother, and I am satisfied would suffer significant harm in the future were he in her care without the making of a care order. The harm would be physical and life-threatening. It seems to me that this is now plainly a case where there is only one way in which the court can properly exercise the discretion conferred under Section 31 of the Children Act, 1989 and I make a care order."

The judge's remark to the effect that courts were not concerned with making a particular diagnosis is worth noting. MSBP carries powerful overtones. The extensive media coverage of the trial and conviction in 1993 of Beverly Allitt of 13 separate offences including murder and attempted murder, committed whilst she suffered from MSBP, may have led to a tendency to think that cases in which MSBP features are qualitatively different from others in which equally serious harm has been suffered. This has led, in some cases, to an insufficiently rigorous approach to controlling the proceedings, and in particular the expert evidence. It is not surprising that the one of the leading cases on the necessity of courts taking control of the proceedings and limiting the expert evidence involved MSBP. In *Re G (Minors)(Expert Witnesses)* [1994] 2 FLR 291, Mr Justice Wall set out in considerable detail the way in which timetables should be set for local authority assessments, a specific expert or area of expertise should be identified when giving leave to disclose papers to an expert, and "the court should, whatever possible, go on to give further directions as to the timescale, the disclosure of the report to the parties and other experts, discussions between experts and the filing of further statements. If it was impracticable to give these directions at the time that leave was granted, the court should set a further date for directions." It was stressed that advocates must apply their minds at an early stage of the case to the issues to which medical evidence would be relevant, and apply for disclosure of the papers as early as possible. The judge reiterated his remarks made in the case of *In Re M* (*Minors*) (*Care Proceedings*) (*Child's Wishes*) [1994] 1 FLR 749 to the effect that experts should always be invited to confer with each other before the final hearing in an attempt to reach agreement or limit the issues, and careful co-operative planning between the legal advisers to the different parties at an early stage in the preparation for trial should be undertaken to ensure the experts' availability and that they can be called to give evidence in a logical sequence.

Mr Justice Wall also emphasised the non-adversarial nature of children's proceedings and stressed the vital importance of expert evidence in assisting the judge to reach the right solutions, saying that

"It is preferable that parents and other litigants approach cases with as many of the factual issues as possible resolved, where such resolution is possible pre-trial. Efficient preparation and presentation of medical evidence is in my judgment an important part of that process."

Re G (*Minors*)(*Expert Witnesses*) [1994] 2 FLR 291 was a case concerning a two-year-old child suffering from both factitious and induced illness, who was placed in the care of the local authority, although his older half-brother went to live with his father.

COVERT VIDEO SURVEILLANCE ("CVS")

The difficulties in confirming a diagnosis of MSBP have led doctors to use covert video surveillance (CVS) to try to establish evidence of the mother's actions. This has inevitably led to questions about whether such surveillance is ethical and admissible in evidence. In *Re DH (A Minor)(Child Abuse)* [1994] 1 FLR 679, a two-year-old boy was admitted to hospital with an upper respiratory tract infection. When he was alone with his mother in a cubicle, he stopped breathing. The consultant paediatrician suspected MSBP, and after further episodes, the mother and child were transferred to a specialist unit where covert video surveillance was used without telling the mother or seeking the father's permission. There were two more assaults which were recorded on video, and on the second occasion, the mother was clearly seen to place something over her son's face. She was arrested and taken to a police station where she was interviewed. Initially, she denied involvement, but having been shown the video she admitted the final incident only and was charged with two counts of cruelty to a child; she pleaded guilty to the second and was placed on probation for three years with a condition of psychiatric treatment. Following an emergency protection order, proceedings for a care order were commenced and by consent the local authority was granted a succession of interim care orders. The child went to stay with his paternal aunt and then returned to live with the father where he thrived.

As to the ethics of covert video surveillance, the judge (again Mr Justice Wall) took the view that they were a matter for doctors, and it was not for him to express a view. As to the admissibility and forensic value of CVS he said "... the paramount concern is the welfare of the child. The protection afforded to the child by the categorical and incontrovertible discovery of the fact and source of the assaults upon him in a clinical setting and surrounded by clear safeguards designed collectively to prevent him from the risk of serious harm greatly outweighs the temporary damage caused by the observed assault. In my judgment, therefore, if the doctor takes the view that CVS is essential for the treatment of his patient he is entitled to undertake it without parental consent, provided that he is satisfied that there is no risk that his patient will come to any serious harm. Critical to this analysis, however, is the foolproof nature of the monitoring process. I am satisfied that the system operated by the specialist unit was as foolproof as any system devised and operated by human beings can be: that it operated properly in the present case with the result that [the child's] interests were immeasurably served by the truth emerging, and the risk to him of further assaults was eliminated. I have also to say from a purely forensic point of view the nature of the evidence provided is invaluable for a number of reasons. First, it puts the issue of the cause of the child's injuries beyond doubt; secondly it affords an opportunity to observe what the mother did in some detail, and may assist in some cases (a) in providing a basis for the assessment of her motivation, and (b) (by gauging her current reaction to it) in helping to assess the stage in the rehabilitative process the mother has reached; thirdly, by rendering denial impossible it obviates the need to spend substantial time in court hearing and evaluating circumstantial lay evidence and what is often inconclusive medical evidence relating to the assaults. This, of course, is not to say that the end justifies the means. Perpetrators of MSBP, however, are rarely suffering from a definable psychiatric illness, and cases of MSBP where the perpetrator is a convincing, apparently concerned parent are commonplace; it is also a characteristic of the syndrome that the perpetrator persists in denials of what has occurred. It follows that the forensic process is enormously advanced by the categorical evidence produced by CVS."

CONTACT WITH THE PERPETRATOR

Contact with the child whilst court proceedings are pending is likely to be contentious, especially if the application for an interim care order is founded on evidence of significant harm, and suspicion about the cause and likely perpetrator. Grave and complex proceedings are inevitably lengthy. The unfolding of evidence as time passes may well result in the contact arrangements prevailing by the time of final hearing being markedly different to those agreed or ordered when the proceedings were commenced. At the commencement of proceedings in which MSBP is suspected but denied, contact with an apparently devoted mother may well be maintained at a high level as rehabilitation remains a viable option. Caution would dictate that the contact is supervised. The extent to which contact can or should be supervised by the other parent or members of the suspected perpetrator's family is often in issue. However, should compelling evidence about causation of the injuries emerge during the pendency of the proceedings, contact may well be reduced.

An expert opinion to the effect that the perpetrator is not amenable to treatment at all, or not within a time scale acceptable for the child, is likely to result in a substantial reduction in contact as the prospect of rehabilitation becomes extremely remote.

In the absence of agreement, the judge will be asked to make an order setting out the terms on which contact will take place, if at all. At one end of the spectrum which includes the overly anxious parent by whom the child is being "mothered to death", mothers excessively dependant on the child and those genuinely believing that there child is ill ("hypochondriasis by proxy"), are children deeply fond of and attached to their mother who may express a wish to live with her. At the other end are mothers who may be suffering from a psychiatric disorder brought about by accident or illness which may be helped by treatment. Contact should not be ruled out simply because the label "MSBP" has been used.

The case law in this area illustrates the breadth of approach taken by the court for whom the child's welfare remains the paramount consideration. It may well be that once safely placed with a caring parent, as in the case *Re DH (A Minor)(Child Abuse)* [1994] 1 FLR 679, the child's contact with the mother could be maintained, not so that she could play a maternal role, but so that the child would have a memory of her, and so that she would not become a frightening fantasy figure, enabling him to come to terms with what she had done to him and for him to come to know her as a kind and loving figure.

REFERENCES

Kelly, C., Loader, P. (1997). Factitious Disorder by Proxy: The role of child mental health professionals. *Child Psychology Psychiatry Rev.* **2(3)**: 116–124.

CHAPTER 12

Risk Assessment

MARY EMINSON
Consultant Child & Adolescent Psychiatrist,
Bolton Hospitals NHS Trust

INTRODUCTION

Assessing risk in MSBP abuse is a particular challenge because of the indirect presentation (concealed nature) of the abuse and the potentially devastating consequences if mistakes are made in judgement of risk. The ultimate questions to be assessed in this situation are: the risks posed to children if they remain at home and what determines those risks; the short- and long-term outcomes of removal from the family or of remaining at home; the evidence for the success of treatment of abusive parents, and the effects and types of monitoring and review. However, before addressing these questions, it is necessary to clarify the nature of the abuse and the timescale of risk.

Types of Abuse

The terminology in the literature on MSBP reflects the confused state of knowledge about this form of abuse and the limited number of studies which adequately define the relevant parameters. In this chapter, the term is restricted to the situation where a parent induces or invents illness in a child and presents to a health care professional. As a consequence, the first imperative in risk assessment is clarity about what has occurred and confidence that sources consulted are describing a strictly comparable sample of cases.

Clarity about what has occurred refers to whether a parent has:

a) physically harmed their child through direct assault themselves (there being a range of severity from direct major physical assaults, such as suffocation, through assault with less immediate consequences such as tampering with drips or alterations in medication),
b) has induced others to unintentionally harm the child (by fabricating a history which results in repeated or intrusive investigations).

For children with pre-existing physical illness (not induced or invented), there are equivalents where parents interfere with or neglect vital treatment; for children with psychiatric disorders, examples of equivalents may be subjection of the child to intrusive and invalidated treatments, for example repeated injections to counter imagined allergens: such treatments on occasion clearly constitute a physical assault. Other crucial variables of the offence include the age of the child who has been the victim, and whether there is evidence that there are other victims in the family now or in the past.

If there is a lack of clarity about events, the efforts of professionals must be directed initially to the clarification of the abuse, whilst ensuring that child protection is maintained during this period. Once it is evident that one of these types of abuse has occurred, it is necessary to undertake a comprehensive and rigorous assessment of social, psychological and medical aspects of the family in the present and historically: an assessment which will consume substantial resources, but is justified where concealed abuse of this kind is under scrutiny.

Types of Risk

The risks being assessed must also be identified with some precision. Physical risks may be divided into (a) immediate risk to the child's health and (b) more distant risk of physical assault. In both circumstances, the risk may include the categories of direct assault, and fabrication to induce assault by others.

No less significant is the risk of psychological harm, which again may be either an immediate and/or long term risk of:

a) Traumatising effects of acute attacks such as suffocation or poisoning.
b) Psychological effects of repeated and lengthy hospitalisation, investigations and examinations.
c) Psychological effects of disturbed relationships and emotional abuse, that is, the effects of being constantly lied to and lied about, of being declared sick when one is well, of being the subject of one's parents' projections and distorted perceptions, rather than being responded to and observed by a perceptive and sensitive parent.

These different types of harm may all be present and may have been repeated.

SOURCES OF INFORMATION ABOUT RISK

As is emphasised in much that is written about risk assessment, the most important single determinant of future risk is past behaviour, which is the key to a proper evaluation of current and future risk. For this, detailed information is required. There is a particular difficulty about gathering information about the past in MSBP abuse. There are three main reasons for this. First, the heart of the problem is in the inaccurate account of events given by the parent; the purpose of which appears to be either to conceal their own part in the physical harm, or to persuade others to investigate and treat a supposed illness in their child. As noted throughout the literature, this habit of invention, evasion and inaccuracy applies to all areas of the history given by the parent, even when the motivation for the untruth is not apparent. Thus, great patience and effort is required to track down sources of information and corroboration.

Second, the nature of history taking about children's illnesses in most British medical settings relies upon an almost literal assumption that the history comes from the parent and that the parent is telling the truth. Most British doctors in paediatric and general practice have received little training in psychiatry, where it is necessary to record both what the patient says and the way in which it is said, as judged by a trained observer. For psychiatrists, both pieces of information are necessary and useful in drawing conclusions about a patient's condition, and neither account has precedence ("Believe everything the patient says and nothing the patient says."). Unfortunately, many non-mental health professionals find offensive the suggestion that the patient's account (or the parent's account) is no more and no less than the patient's account and may require corroboration from a variety of sources. Many doctors reject this idea as inconsistent with their view of the doctor–patient relationship, as it implies a lack of trust. This problem affects both the way the history is taken and the written notes: these too rarely distinguish the parent's account from the direct observations of the physician or other independent person.

Third, the suggestion of MSBP abuse properly produces great anxiety in professionals, especially hospital nursing and medical teams. These individuals become very concerned to prevent harm to children. As a result, small actions of parents under suspicion may be misconstrued or over-interpreted and the reactions of the staff themselves start to confuse the picture: in other words, the difficulty of separating objective facts and subjective impressions exists in the present observations of the parent as well as in the history.

CONSTRUCTING A RISK ASSESSMENT FROM THE AVAILABLE INFORMATION

Clarity about the risks for any single child rests on an integration of knowledge about their specific situation (summarised into a series of areas of inquiry in Fig. 1) with information from the scientific literature to reach conclusions about each of the domains of potential risk (see Fig. 2). These domains of potential risk are derived from the literature to encapsulate the crucial determining factors for abuse of this type.

INFORMATION FROM THE CURRENT SITUATION

It will be evident then that undertaking risk assessment for MSBP requires a meticulous examination not only of the patient, the parent and

Area of inquiry	Source of information
Child's current state of health.	GP, hospital reports.
Health of parent, and health care seeking behaviour by parent.	Parent's own account, GP and hospital records, other family members' accounts.
Relationships between parent and child, parent and partner, parent and professional.	Direct observation. Report of main partner. Experience of all other professionals.
Social circumstances.	HV, GP and social work records.
Parent's mental state and personality.	Direct observation. GP and hospital records. Expert view needed on occasion.
Current behaviour towards child and current relationship with child. Current behaviour between all family members. (Measurable and recordable acts)	Direct observation. Report of health professional as judged by trained enquirer - ward nurses - medical staff - HV, GP, social worker - other family members.
Family relationships and functioning, subjective and objective, past and present (emotions, patterns of relationships).	Family members' own account. Direct observation, including mental health specialists and other observers.
Parent's life story: this includes physical health, social, educational and legal aspects.	Parent's own account, plus accounts from relatives, partners and other records.
History of illness and illness behaviour in the whole family.	GP, HV, hospital and school records.
History of abuse or contact with social services.	Social workers' records, GP and HV records. Records of case conferences.
Child's previous health and development. History of development of other children.	GP and HV records. Hospital records and school reports.
History of parent's mental state.	GP and hospital records. Family reports.
History of engagement with professional help of all kinds.	Record scrutiny and account of professionals with longest contact with family.

Fig. 1.   Areas of risk inquiry.

Domains of potential risk
• Extent and nature of harm which has already occurred.
• Mental health, personality and cognitive ability of parent.
• Capacity to form trusting relationships characterised by openness and honesty.
• Acknowledgement of what has occurred.
• Capacity to use professional help in order to change.
• Capacity to distinguish child's needs from own.
• Formulation of family patterns, strengths and weaknesses.
• Extent of available family support to ensure safety, child protection, and assist change.
• Extent of professional network to monitor and/or assist in treatment.

Fig. 2.   Domains of potential risk.

the current events, but that scrutiny of the history may require direct examination of the primary sources: original hospital and primary care and GP records (which may give clues to concealed changes of name and address), social services records and often, assessment of all individuals of relevance including the partner and family members of any abusive parent whose risk is being assessed. Different professionals may be required in this assessment, because different expertise is required in different areas. Although local professionals usually contribute most of the information, other professional views may be needed to come to conclusions about certain domains of risk.

Space does not permit the discussion of these domains of risk in any detail, but these are in any case the types of assessments which form the bedrock of child protection. What is unusual is the need to integrate the appraisal of medical presentations into the social and psychological assessments, rather than the somewhat separate reports possible in physical and sexual abuse cases. This demands sophisticated and detailed scrutiny of notes and on occasion, careful discussion between health care professionals, to assess whether presentations in health care have been due to intrinsic conditions, factitious symptoms, or where this truly cannot be resolved. The family assessment too must be a sophisticated one which results in an analysis of possible aetiological factors and, crucially, of the potential for protection in future. Finally, the assessment of the parent who has perpetrated the abuse must be one which takes a broad view including childhood, adolescent and adult functioning (including the possibility of obstetric factitious symptoms).

With these considerations taken into account the good and poor prognostic indicators in these domains are as in any child protection assessment: severity and chronicity of harm, extensive personality and forensic problems, evidence of widespread dissembling, abuse in other children, persistent denial in parent or partner, failure to develop trust or be able to explore the consequences of the abuse for the child victim and lack of an adequate professional network must all be considered to raise risk and concern.

SOURCES OF INFORMATION: THE SCIENTIFIC LITERATURE

Once detailed information about the particular family has been acquired, this can be combined with information from other cases as available from published sources. The scientific literature here may be summarised under one of the following headings:

1. Clinical Series where MSBP Abuse has been Recognised

These studies are the most substantial source of information on risk. The various studies of Meadow and his co-workers, Bools and Neale, are some of the most systematic in their evaluation of a cohort of children and parents identified over a long period (Meadow, 1985; 1991). Comorbidity in other family members as well as outcomes for children returned and removed, have been studied in this group of families (Bools, Neale and Meadow, 1992; 1993; 1994). Meadow (1985) initially described six factors as "most worrying" from a paediatric viewpoint:

i) severe abuse (i.e., a severe physical assault, either direct or indirect)
ii) abuse of a child under five years
iii) previous unexplained sibling deaths

iv) lack of acknowledgement of the behaviour of the parent or lack of explanation if the parent makes some form of acknowledgement

v) parents with Munchausen Syndrome (because of the deception involved), and substance abuse

vi) persistence of fabrication even after confrontation

The risks of other assaults upon the index child, and the risks to other family members prior to the index fabrication are examined in Bools, Neale and Meadow's study of 56 children and 82 of their 103 siblings (1992). Forty one (73%) of the index children suffered abuse other than the index fabrication: this included other fabrications, failure to thrive, non-accidental injury, inappropriate medication or neglect. Although the records of siblings were incomplete, 39% (40 children from 26 families) had also been the subject of fabricated illness, 17% (18) had suffered failure to thrive, non-accidental injury, inappropriate medication or neglect. Thirteen siblings had died; overall, 43% of siblings (from 29 of the 43 families studied) were affected by abuse. The authors link the high morbidity rates to the severity of abuse in their index cases, more than half having suffered direct physical abuse (suffocation, poisoning or skin abrasions). Thus, the evidence is that where early severe direct physical abuse has occurred, there is a long term risk of similar difficulties including deaths in vulnerable children in such households. Two further British series confirm the risks to siblings in households where early direct physical harm has occurred. Southall et al.'s (1997) series of 33 suffocations (or similar) confirmed on covert video surveillance contains reports of 12 sibling deaths. McClure et al.'s (1996) series of 128 cases (suffocations, poisonings and fabricated histories) has 83 families with siblings, of which 34 had suffered previous abuse; in the entire cohort there had been 18 previous sibling deaths.

2. Children Remaining in MSBP Abusive Households after Identification of Fabrications

Whilst the data in this study is admittedly incomplete, Bools, Neale and Meadow's (1993) follow-up of the 30 children from their original series, who continued to live with their mothers after the index fabrication, remains the most substantive available. Of the 18 children for whom they had adequate data, 13 were judged to have significant disorders judged by clinical interview with family members, screening questionnaires and information from schools. Further fabrications had occurred in ten children, of whom seven suffered a psychiatric disorder. Thus, the outcomes for these children were poor both in terms of short-term physical health, short-term psychological and educational functioning and longer-term adjustment. Three fifths (12/21) had what were described as unacceptable outcomes. The extent of subsequent monitoring was crucial.

In a more recent study (Davis *et al.*, 1998) 39 children were followed up for 12–22 months after return home following child protection registrations for abuse via fabricated histories (i.e., parents inducing doctors to commit the harm). No children suffering suffocations or poisonings are included. As measured by the reports of paediatricians, in two children further fabrication occurred, three suffered emotional abuse, one received physical abuse (15%). These children were subjected to a variety of monitoring conditions.

3. Children Removed from MSBP Abusive Households

The Leeds follow-up study (Bools, Neale and Meadow, 1993) also examined 24 children removed following fabrications. As already noted, their cohort included a high proportion of severe assaults including smothering and many of the most severely assaulted young children were removed. Several of the nine smothered children had particular short-term, emotional problems which appeared to be reactions to the smothering experience. Overall, children who had been removed were younger than those who remained within abusive households and three fifths (12) had acceptable outcomes in terms of emotional, physical and educational development. In the same study, 54 children were followed up 1 to 14 years after identification of fabrications. Psychological aspects of harm (including emotional, physical and educational development) were examined. Risks of adverse outcomes in these domains were associated with long delays before intervention, and multiple placements in care.

The authors acknowledge that these careful studies include children of varied ages and perhaps more importantly, who had experienced abuse of different kinds (severe and less severe physical assault and fabrications to induced assault by others). This heterogeneity increases the difficulty of establishing risks for those who do not possess the major indicators of poor prognosis for both short- and long-term emotional and physical development (early, severe, prolonged abuse with severe comorbidity, and severe social disruption).

Rosenberg (1987) comments on the "few remarks relating to the psychiatric follow-up" of the 107 survivors in her early literature review, including a very few identified as demonstrating long-term psychological sequelae; sparse reports are likely to be due simply to a lack of assessment of the relevant parameters.

4. Clinical Accounts of Treatment Interventions where Harm has Occurred

A limited number of case reports and descriptive accounts of treatment interventions have been published from a variety of theoretical perspectives (Nicol and Eccles, 1985; Loader and Kelly, 1996; Jones et al., 2000); the last two being descriptions of inpatient programmes; these emphasise the central importance of full perpetrator acknowledgement of the abuse if treatment towards safe return home is to be achieved. Obviously less severe cases are selected for outpatient work even if the child is not at home when this takes place. The processes involved in treatment of the perpetrator, child and family differ in these accounts not least in the amount of intervention but the essential elements in all seem to be ending denial; exploration of the perpetrator's own early life to help acknowledging and understanding their past abusive experiences; development of parenting skills; an actively protective stance from other family members; development of alternative strategies for managing stressful circumstances and continued close monitoring and support. Anecdotally, for those who can remain engaged with professionals whilst these tasks are completed, the outlook is positive. Only a minority of selected cases will even be considered for such an approach. These descriptions are helpful in that the detail assists in deciding where cases are matched on the significant variables. These must be carefully scrutinised before drawing conclusions about risk in analogous circumstances.

5. Child Abuse Literature

The extensive general child abuse literature (Cicchetti and Lynch, 1995) allows more confidence about predicting outcomes where the categorisation of abuse is very similar to that in MSBP. In particular, the outcomes for children are likely to be highly generalisable from these series. Generally, many variables found in MSBP abuse (the concealed nature of the abuse, all the problems of engaging with the perpetrator on therapeutic endeavours, the difficulties the offending parents have in making trusting relationships generally) are poor prognostic indicators. This literature is particularly helpful in the area of physical abuse where the factors which indicate high risk for re-occurrence (Cicchetti and Lynch, 1995), both immediately and later, are virtually identical to those derived from the MSBP literature. For early, severe physically harmful abuse (suffocations, poisonings) the outcomes from these series are likely to be highly generalisable to MSBP abuse circumstances.

Many studies now also integrate developmental considerations into both evaluation of risk and examination of outcomes (Cicchetti and Toth, 1995) and treatment. This approach is particularly helpful when evaluating risk and drawing up child protection plans in MSBP abuse situations of fabricated illness and inventions of symptoms in older children. These are likely to be circumstances of lesser levels of physical harm and with positive indicators in the other domains of risk.

6. Adult Mental Health Literature about Risks to Children of Parents with Mental Impairments or Ill Health

The majority of MSBP abusive parents do not suffer from clear mental illness but do suffer from personality difficulties often with accompanying depression, anxiety and substance abuse (Bools *et al.*, 1994). Such parents have well recognised difficulties in relationships with their children, as with professionals. The potential outcomes for their children in terms of emotional and behavioural difficulties, even if MSBP abuse is not evident, have been recognised (Norton and Dolan, 1996; Seeman, 1996). These findings are rarely so specific as to be helpful in prognosis for the individual case, but are useful when integrated with other information about family strengths and functioning, available support and monitoring capacities, and evidence of potential for containing the abusive parent's behaviour and/or agreement in therapeutic work.

Oates (1997) recently reviewed the risk of all forms of parental mental illness for children. Whilst the individual studies examined in this review are rarely controlled and the measures for children's outcomes vary in their level of sophistication, nevertheless, this literature may be particularly helpful in risk assessment where the abusing parent does have an identifiable mental illness, the effect of which explains some or all of their abusive behaviour. Overall, the adult mental health literature also serves to reinforce the impression that the presence of other non-abusive, actively protective and abuse acknowledging adults in the family is a crucial protective factor.

Of course, vitrually all MSBP cases constitute severe emotional abuse alongside physical risks and for the majority of those who survive the physical assaults this may be the most substantial long-term risk (Ney, 1994). Chronic somatisation and other mental health problems including self harm, difficulty in forming trusting relationships, poor parenting skills, must be long-term vulnerabilities of this group, as indeed they are the risk factors for its occurrence.

CONCLUSIONS

The recognition of this severe form of abuse comes at a time when research is ongoing into the outcomes for children of all types of parental abuse. Uncertainties of definition of abuse have contributed. We are still at an early stage, however, in identifying appropriate actions to remediate the effects or to plan treatments. This is especially true where the abuse involves fabrications only and where immediate permanent removal does not appear to be the only safe course. It is in these circumstances that the conclusions drawn about the various domains of risk must carry the greatest weight and must therefore be made with enormous care. There is however nothing magical or mysterious about how the risks are weighed. Such decisions will normally be made by integrating the assessments of many people, incorporating much information about the longitudinal pattern of individuals' and families' functioning, and including the weight of child protection legal systems.

If, following risk assessment, the decision has been made to undertake a period of monitoring and intervention for a family, a clear, precise plan is necessary. This includes a timescale for review and clear identification of the indicators of good and poor progress. This may determine the extent of risk for the period after the abuse has been recognised. Just as the risk assessment at the time of identification can only be made with good information, so the continuing risk assessment rests on the quality of monitoring information. This should include the original domains of risk, but should be far more precise as the crucial variables for this family are now known. The involvement of all relevant professionals from different disciplines is more important in these cases than in almost any other. Their close co-operation, shared understanding and good communication are essential. Involvement of primary care professionals, who are the gatekeepers to further sets of medical referrals and are aware of parental stresses and somatic presentations, is a frequent lacuna in this respect.

A need clearly remains for more studies of the long-term outcomes of MSBP victims and perpetrators, including both social and psychological measures of families whether remaining together with treatment or where separation has occurred. Except for that small number of families who are involved in a detailed residential assessment (Jones, 2000) decisions about keeping families together will largely depend on the extent of available local professional networks in social services, health (primary and secondary care, mental and physical) and education. These networks will need to monitor closely and to offer appropriate treatment for parents and children as their existing skills and resources permit (Loader and Kelly, 1996; Nicol and Eccles, 1985). In the majority of circumstances, the patterns of difficulties which precipitates MSBP abuse are severe and chronic ones and the monitoring and treatment interventions also need to have this perspective: one which implies the commitment of resources for a long period.

REFERENCES

Bools, C. N., Neale, B. A., Meadow, S. R. (1992). Co-morbidity associated with fabricated illness (Munchausen Syndrome by Proxy). *Arch. Dis. Child.* **67**: 77–79.

Bools, C., Neale, B., Meadow, S. R. (1994). Munchausen Syndrome by Proxy: Study of psychopathology. *Child Abuse Negl.* **18**: 773–788.

Bools, C., Neale, B., Meadow, S. R. (1993). Follow up of victims of fabricated illness (Munchausen Syndrome by Proxy). *Arch. Dis. Child.* **69**: 625–630.

Cicchetti, D., Lynch, M. (1995). Failures in the expectable environment and their impact on individual development: The case of child maltreatment. In: *Developmental Psychopathology*, eds. Cicchetti, D. and Cohen, D. (Wiley, London) **2**: 32–72.

Cicchetti, D., Toth, S. L. (1995). A developmental psychopathology perspective on child abuse and neglect. *J. Am. Acad. Child. Adolesc. Psychiatry* **34(5)**: 541–565.

Davis, P., McClure, R. J., Chessman, N., Pearson, S., Sibert, J. R., Meadow, R. (1998). Procedures, placement, and risks of further abuse after Munchausen Syndrome by Proxy, non-accidental poisoning, and non-accidental suffocation. *Arch. Dis. Child.* **78**: 217–221.

Eminson, D. M., Postlethwaite, R. J. (1992). Factitious illness: Recognition and management. *Arch. Dis. Child.* **67**: 1510–1516.

Gray, J., Bentovim, A. (1996). Illness induction syndrome: Paper 1. A series of 41 children from 37 families identified at the Great Ormond Street Hospital for Children NHS Trust. *Child Abuse Negl.* **20(8)**: 655–673.

Jones, D. (2000). Management, treatment and outcomes. In: *Munchausen Syndrome by Proxy Abuse. A practical approach*, eds. Eminson, D. M. and Postlethwaite, R. J. (Butterworth, Heinemann).

Loader, P., Kelly, C. (1996). Munchausen Syndrome by Proxy: A narrative approach to explanation. *Clin. Psych. Psychol.* **1(3)**: 353–363.

McGuire, T. L., Feldman, K. W. (1989). Psychological morbidity of children subjected to Munchausen Syndrome by Proxy. *Pediatrics* **83**: 289–292.

Meadow, R. (1985). Management of Munchausen Syndrome by Proxy. *Arch. Dis. Child.* **60**: 385–393.

Nicol, A. R., Eccles, M. (1985). Psychotherapy for Munchausen Syndrome by Proxy. *Arch. Dis. Child.* **60**: 385–393.

Oates, M. R. (1997). Patients as parents: The risk to children. *Br. J. Psych.* **170(32)**(suppl.): 22–27.

Ney, P. (1994). The worst combinations of child abuse and neglect. *Child Abuse Negl.* **18**: 707–714.

Norton, K., Dolan, B. (1996). Personality disorder and parenting. In: *Parental Psychiatric Disorder: Distressed Parents and their Families*, eds. Göpfert, Webster and Seeman. (Cambridge University Press, Cambridge) 219–232.

Pound, A. (1996). Parental affective disorder in childhood disturbance. In: *Parental Psychiatric Disorder: Distressed Parents and their Families*, eds. Göpfert, Webster and Seeman. (Cambridge University Press, Cambridge) 201–218.

Rosenberg, D. A. (1987). Web of deceit: A literature review of Munchausen Syndrome by Proxy. *Child Abuse Negl.* **11**: 547–563.

Seeman, M. V. (1996). The mother with schizophrenia. In: *Parental Psychiatric Disorder: Distressed Parents and their Families*, eds. Göpfert, Webster and Seeman. (Cambridge University Press, Cambridge) 190–220.

Southall, D. P., Plunkett, C. B., Banks, M. W., Falkov, A. F., Samuels, M. P. (1997). Covert video recordings of life-threatening child abuse: Lessons for child protection. *Pediatrics* **100(5)**: 735–760.

CHAPTER 13

Treatment of Perpetrators

KERRY BLUGLASS

Consultant Psychiatrist,
Woodbourne Priory Hospital, Birmingham,
Senior Clinical Lecturer, University of Birmingham

INTRODUCTION

Early case reports of characteristics of "MSBP" parents described the most severe, striking and dangerous or potentially dangerous acts of parents towards their children, and usually characterised them as having severe personality disorders. Clinicians therefore usually assumed that no treatment was appropriate or possible, and were pessimistic about favourable outcomes or the likelihood of reunification of the parent and child. With the growing importance of detailed psychiatric assessment of the parents, we are beginning to recognise the wide diversity of parental characteristics and behaviours. With this recognition, we have come to understand that exploration of the circumstances and mental state of the individual sometimes reveals a parent or parents where possibilities exist for future change. It is important to distinguish between such capacity to change and benefit from therapeutic intervention as an individual and that which may also lead to the possibility of reunification with the child or children as a safe or "good enough" parent, within a timescale which is appropriate for the child(ren) and which does not result in an interminable delay.

ASSESSMENT

Assessment of the family as a whole is essential, but it is useful to consider first the factors involved in the behaviour of the parent implicated in the aberrant illness behaviour by detailed investigation. Traditionally we have used the outpatient consultation, often based on several interviews. There are usually no facilities for inpatient assessment unless so ordered by the courts. However recently we have developed a short, intensive assessment programme for mothers. Where appropriate the parent(s) may later proceed to a later family assessment — sometimes with a possible view to treatment at specialised units which have particular expertise in this field.

Legal aid may assist the funding of the assessment of the mother in this general psychiatric unit. We have commonly seen the presentation of a mother, sometimes dominated by a forceful or unsupportive partner, who is unable to express herself or her own needs, who has a history of illness behaviour, or who seeks relief from anxiety over a child who is sick, or is perceived to be so, through paediatric consultations. Often this has led to one or more admissions to a paediatric ward.

Improved recognition and diagnosis has resulted in better management, and although denial is common initially, some of our referrals have admitted already to inducing illness or factitiously claiming symptoms. During the assessment we then concentrate on exploring their motivation and promoting better understanding of their behaviour. Alternatively, the mother may acknowledge a need for personal help, given that child care proceedings are in progress, but may have made no admission or only a partial one. It is no part of the assessment process to "extract confession", but to focus on the needs of the individual parent, in order to begin to understand the context of what is alleged. This may initiate a process which paves the way for a more prolonged and family-based intervention, either on an outpatient basis or by progression to an inpatient assessment/treatment facility at units such as the Park Hospital, Oxford (see Chapter by Jones) or the Cassel Hospital, Richmond (Kennedy, 1997). In other cases, appropriate treatment in the community has been arranged and in well-selected cases appears to be working well.

We are now beginning to see the fruits of such collaborative assessment/ treatment endeavours with reunification in some cases. Clearly the very long-term follow-up results of such work are not yet available, but will be extremely important. Success rates at present quoted by such units appear to be of the order of 40%, which of course relates only to a carefully selected group. Even where a team makes no recommendation for direct family work leading to restoration of the child(ren) to the parents with any likelihood of success, the assessment process can do much to help the parent(s) to understand the reasoning behind the decisions of the court, to express their distress, anger and feelings of loss (whether short- or long-term), and also to diminish or identify any risk to future children or the community. Sometimes, the parent(s) may appear to be suitable for rehabilitation/reunification but the child may be too damaged emotionally, either by the original abuse or by the inevitable separation and period of time in care, to be able to wait for an uncertain outcome of treatment of the parent(s). Here, part of the further work with the family involves trying to help the process of adjustment to this decision. As part of the assessment process, some of us are now engaged in collaborative research into the attachment characteristics of these parents, and hope to improve further identification of those in whom intervention is likely to be successful.

TREATMENT AND INTERVENTION

We now recognise that the psychopathology, mental states, intellectual ability and maturity of parents suspected of involvement in factitious or induced illnesses in children vary enormously, and the variation in motivation and intent is similarly diverse. Looking at the cases described in the United States of America, particularly in the work of Libow and Schreier (1986), the severity of the behaviours they describe is striking, and in fact they doubt the wide variation, indicating that in their opinion, almost all forms of this behaviour, if correctly classified as Munchausen Syndrome by Proxy are necessarily extremely dangerous. There is still of course a pressing need for diagnostic rigour in this area.

In the United Kingdom, there is now, as a consequence of these and other authors' timely warnings, an increasing degree of awareness — particularly since the reporting of a recent dramatic case of a nurse who caused deaths and illness of several children. As a result, the "label" now seems to us to be almost over-used and certainly misunderstood — for example, by legal representatives of some parents who may believe that if proven, this "disorder" of the parent(s) will result in mitigation. Clearly much professional education is required. Our impression therefore, in the United Kingdom, is that the spectrum of severity concept is useful, but we should not however ignore the need to describe and evaluate behaviour since, as discussed, intent may be highly dangerous despite an apparently "minor" action, and vice versa (a dangerous act not perceived as such by the parent).

Rarely do parents admit to a murderous intent, although of course children do indeed die in fatal forms of this abuse, but markedly ambivalent attitudes often emerge on exploration of the parent's history. As is the case with suicide, attempted or completed, the intention can therefore fail in either direction due to the perpetrator's inadequate knowledge of the likely consequences of the behaviour. Thus, severity of the intent cannot always be directly inferred from the behaviour. This is important to consider when assessing risk.

Since there is now enormously increased recognition by child protection teams and paediatricians, we receive regular requests to assess and treat, or refer for treatment, mothers who have already admitted to a partial or full extent their involvement in their child's illness. The "explanation" given in such acknowledgement may be a partial or superficial one, but it seems to be generally agreed that accepting responsibility in this way is at least a starting point for any consideration of therapeutic work which may lead to consideration of rehabilitation. Conversely, continued denial or apportioning blame to others usually confines any work to an investigative or exploratory level. Sometimes it may be possible to engage the parent in some form of therapeutic process by an agreed mutual acknowledgement that, by virtue of involvement in the child protection proceedings, the family is facing considerable strains. In criminal proceedings, the parent is often inaccessible to intervention until after their completion. Even after a custodial sentence, in some circumstances, however, effective work may result in family reunification through psychotherapeutic intervention, and I have seen significant work begun in custody with subsequent reunification, still apparently successful at two-year follow-up.

Since Meadow (1977) first described the syndrome (MSBP) reports of treatment approaches have been hard to find. Initially, only the most severe and obvious behaviours were identified and it was therefore not surprising that clinicians seldom considered therapeutic intervention, especially since the most striking finding in perpetrators were incorrigible forms of personality; narcissistic, histrionic and manipulative, frequently with poor differentiation of their own boundaries and needs from those of their children. Schreier and Libow (1993) in their comprehensive text freely acknowledge the pessimistic overview which the literature and their own experience indicates and rightly question the motivation of some parents to accept treatment if it is simply directed at "eluding the protective services and accelerating the return of their children." They warn against a notional therapeutic endeavour if it is superficial, insufficiently frequent and/or performed by a therapist "unfamiliar with the powerful dynamics these parents present." This is why in my own recommendations in court, I am personally very cautious unless I can be reassured about the competence and experience of the proposed therapist. A "counsellor" already engaged in working with the mother on the loss of her children to child protection proceedings, foster care, where the mother sees herself as the injured party, or only on issues of her own past trauma — even though these may be legitimate issues — will not suffice as challenging and aware therapist in this context. Forensically trained and experienced clinicians familiar with the range of personality and borderline disorders are less likely to be manipulated or seduced by the possible distortions of some of these parents in treatment.

Nicol and Eccles (1985) described a successful treatment outcome with psychotherapy. More recently, Black and Hollis (1996) considered that "with careful case selection and modifications to treatment approaches, the generally poor prognosis might be improved." They reported the details of the treatment of a family over ten systemic therapy sessions with successful follow-up at four years.

The absence of other published reports of promising therapy does not mean that it has not occurred and clinicians should consider disseminating their experience, even of single cases.

Essentially therefore any consideration of treatment begins with a formulation based on a careful assessment of the individual at a clinical level including the usual detailed scrutiny of the general practice and other medical notes, usually already available for the purpose of reporting to the court, whether for child protection or criminal proceedings. A "forensic" approach appropriate for assessment of any abusive or offending behaviour helps the clinician to preserve an objective stance.

Where a finding of frank mental disorder is made, any treatment plan should obviously consider the relief of that illness. By definition hitherto undetected delusional symptoms are unlikely to be present, since an obvious psychotic illness would take diagnostic priority. In practice, although post natal depression is often cited as a possible mechanism and may be a contributory factor, as a single explanation I have not found it to be common either in my own or colleagues' series of cases. Nevertheless, its detection clearly forms a vital part of the assessment, as does the existence of other disorder such as obsessional or eating disorders, or substance abuse.

In our practice, a full multi-disciplinary assessment during a two-week inpatient stay also allows the parent, in a non-judgmental setting, the opportunity to begin to appreciate more appropriate ways of managing stress, anger, help seeking, and self expression, and to begin to understand and acknowledge the interplay of family and marital relationships, with particular application to the welfare and care of the child(ren) in the nuclear and extended family. This initial process may provide a step towards a full family assessment/intervention process which is itself a step-wise procedure (see Jones, 2000).

THE TREATMENT AND INTERVENTION PROCESS

Professional Good Practice

Parnell and Day (1997), from their perspective in providing opinions for court proceedings and treatment for perpetrators, have reviewed the relatively sparse literature on these issues, rightly emphasising the distinctive roles of professionals. Once significant therapeutic work is undertaken, issues of confidentiality and trust are fundamental to the process. Revelations of detail (for example, to other professionals or to the courts concerned with progress or risk assessments) can only be made with the agreement of the patient/parent. Welldon (1996) has discussed the dilemmas posed by such interactions for the professional engaged in forensic work. Other equally important matters such as burn-out, co-therapists (Parnell and Day, ibid) and supervision (Bluglass, 1996; Welldon, 1996) require careful consideration, particularly when the proliferation of assessment/treatment requests now increasingly involves professionals with little or no previous experience in such work.

In addition to good professional practice and the mutually supportive functions of seminars, conferences and other educational activities, we find it useful to organise informal clinical peer support meetings between those engaged in the treatment of similar or overlapping cases, to enhance practice and draw on a wider range of experience. Whilst individual professional supervision will address issues such as transference, splitting, manipulation, over-involvement with some of these extremely complex, convincing and often seductive personalities, peer support and review is effective in highlighting some of the emerging dynamic problems and hitherto unconsidered difficulties. As Day (1998) remarks in relation to co-therapists (the later therapeutic stage: identity reformation) "having clinical feedback from another therapist who is familiar with the facts of the case will also provide the therapist with a way to measure success with a patient. The less he or she has to confer with the co-therapist and the less 'crazy' he or she feels, the better the case is going."

Whilst there is almost universal recognition that prospects of successful treatment are as slim or non-existent with those perpetrators with severe personality disorders as they would be for other offenders or abusers, it should not encourage therapeutic nihilism towards more malleable individuals who may respond. Defining those parents in whom a measure of successful outcome has been achieved is an important a part of our work, and long-term follow-up studies will be essential, not least because of the indications of long-term sequelae for some of the affected children (McGuire and Feldman, 1989; Bools, Neal and Meadow, 1993).

Expectations of Treatment

I have emphasised the importance of trying to determine, as early as possible in the assessment process, the important distinction between those perpetrators who would benefit from psychotherapeutic intervention for themselves (and wider family, community, non-abused and possible future children or other potential recipients of their care — including residents of homes or institutions where they might seek employment), and those where the ability to function as "good enough" parent is an achievable goal, on the other. Since some of these parents have many unresolved and sometimes undisclosed personal problems, such as physical, emotional and/or sexual abuse, eating and other disorders, as with other patients who receive psychotherapeutic and other specialised interventions, it is reasonable to try to address these. The courts and other professionals, especially defence lawyers, should be aware when such intervention is a recommendation for the individual only and carries no guarantee of a likely reunification with the index child (or siblings), ever, or within a foreseeable timescale without further uncertainty of a stable placement for the child.

Sometimes either the diagnostic or legal processes have been so protracted that the child(ren) have been in alternative care for so long that the prospect of a further delay to initiate and evaluate therapeutic work may be unacceptable. The therapist may then have to work not only with the past and present dynamic issues, but with aspects of guilt, loss, anger and recrimination, whilst trying to enable the parent(s) to move forward towards better future functioning in all dimensions of their lives, including potential parenting.

Treatment Methods

The detail of treatment where such diverse motivations and personality factors are involved clearly has to be formulated on an individual case basis, and in this sense is no different from the planning of intervention for any form of offending or abusive behaviour. Additional constraints of time planning, needs of the child(ren) for contact, further reports to court and other agencies, are specialised aspects of the work. This is broadly psychotherapy with a special focus, and of course a range of modalities including cognitive behavioural therapy and family therapy may be required. A need for the patient to mature, to acknowledge the harm (actual and potential) done to the child, to differentiate between his/her own needs and the child's in order to put the latter before the former, to relinquish denial and blaming others as defensive strategies, and to learn to seek help and self expression in appropriate ways, are the goals of treatment. Surrounding issues of family, marital, personal and financial as well as vocational problems must be included.

Day and Parnell (ibid); Day (ibid); and Day and Ojeda-Castro (Parnell and Day, ibid) have divided the process, including the setting up of the treatment framework, and three stages (initial, middle and later) which provide a clear and thoughtful model of the special nature of the therapeutic work involved, which will be invaluable for workers in the field . They frequently acknowledge the difficulties and hazards encountered in this work. Their experience should be obligatory study for those embarking on treatment of these individuals and families.

Black and Hollis (ibid) considered the following good prognostic signs in their case to be

1. acknowledgement of the abuse,
2. good family support,
3. a willingness to work with professional helpers,
4. the presence of specific stressors at the time.

They also highlighted some caveats, including the lack of admission of illlness induction in anolder child and some lack of sensitivity to the suffering of a tiny baby.

We all have an obligation to audit, review and disseminate our therapeutic successes and failures, particularly in long-term follow-up, in order to provide the best possible service for the protection of children and the provision of intervention for those parents likely to respond to it. The pendulum of therapeutic possibility should not swing from the wholly negative to the unrealistically over-optimistic, but we should bear in mind the spirit and principles of the Children Act, ensuring fundamental protection for the child, where possible in his/her family of origin.

REFERENCES

Bluglass, K. (1996). *A Practical Guide to Forensic Psychotherapy*, eds. Welldon, E. and Van van Velsen, C. (Kingsley Publishers, London).

Black, D., Hollis, P. J. (1996). *Child Psychol. Psychiatry* **1**: 89–98.

Bools, C. N., Neale, B. A., Meadow, S. R. (1993). Follow up of victims of fabricated illness (MSBP). *Arch. Dis. Child.* **69**: 625–630.

Jones, David P. H., Newbold, Caroline (2000). Assessment of abusing families. In *Muchausen's Syndrome by Proxy*, eds. Adshead, Gwen and Brooke, Deborah, Chapter 8 (Imperial College Press, London).

Kennedy, R. (1997). *Child Abuse, Psychotherapy and the Law.* Free Association Books.

Libow, J. A., Schreier, H. A. (1986). *Am. J. Orthopsychiatry* **56**: 602–611.

McGuire, T. L., Feldman, N. D. (1989). Psychological morbidity of children subjected to Munchausen Syndrome by Proxy. *Paediatrics* **83**: 289–292.

Meadow, R. (1977). *Lancet* **2**: 343–345.

Nicol, A. R., Eccles, M. (1985). *Arch. Dis. Child.* **60**: 344–348.

Ojeda-Castro, M. D. (1998). *Munchausen by Proxy Syndrome*, eds. Parnell, T. F. and Day, D. O. (Sage, London, New York).

Parnell, T. F., Day, D. O. (1998). *Munchausen by Proxy Syndrome* (Sage, London, New York).

Schreier, H. A., Libow, J. A. (1993). *Hurting for Love.* (Guilford Press, London and New York).

CHAPTER 14

Treatment and Outcome for Victims

IAN MITCHELL

Professor, Department of Paediatrics &
Head of Paediatric Respirology,
University of Calgary

GENERAL ISSUES

If Munchausen Syndrome by Proxy (MSBP) was truly a disease, then this chapter, with accepted and proven treatments and a list of consequences of the treated and untreated "disease" would be both essential and straightforward. Yet some would consider MSBP a descriptor of an unusual form of child abuse rather than a disease (Emminson *et al.*, 1992; Fisher and Mitchell, 1995). If it is a disease, it is one of parent/child relationships, not a disease of a parent alone, and certainly not one of the child alone. However, the traditional word "disease" will be used in this chapter, without being too specific as to who has the disease! In such a complex and confused situation, the word "treatment" is used to describe an overall management strategy in which many different professionals are involved. Thus, treatment must start the moment the diagnosis is considered, not when it is proven, and it must be long-term. The professionals involved include paediatricians and family physicians (and often specialist paediatricians), nurses, social workers, psychologists, child psychiatrists, lawyers, police, child protection authorities and so on, and must work as a team. Such a diverse multi-disciplinary team, with different professional and personal philosophies dealing with a variety of medical, social and psychological problems, will need to consider many different treatment objectives and often will have to make choices between them. For example, some team members may focus entirely on the child's protection, others will want preservation of the family as their main objective, and others still will focus on issues of guilt, innocence or punishment. A management plan should be developed by consensus but treatment objectives must be clear. Regular communication between team members is essential to ensure continuing consensus, and clarity of objectives, as circumstances change.

Knowledge of outcomes is used in paediatrics to guide effective treatment, but in MSBP such information is scanty. The information that is available is alarming, in terms of death and handicap. Moreover, the outcome when the diagnosis is not made is worse and may include death. In MSBP, as in any other child abuse situation, the whole family must be considered in treatment plans and descriptions of outcomes. The sibling must be given detailed attention. Southall *et al.* (1997) is only one of many authors who report the possibility of abuse, and sometimes even death in siblings. The earlier the diagnosis of MSBP is considered, the earlier it can be confirmed or refuted. Diagnosis is the responsibility of the paediatrician. In too many cases the diagnosis is not considered because: it is not known to the physicians; it is known but is perceived to be rare; or it is explored only after all alternative physical illnesses have been disproven. Education can deal with some of these problems, but the last is deeply rooted in medical and institutional culture and is more difficult to eradicate. In paediatrics generally, the relationship between parents and paediatrician is important and positive, but in the case of MSBP this positive relationship may itself delay identification of the underlying causes of the child's illness. The diagnosis of MSBP should be considered whenever it seems a possible explanation for the clinical situation. MSBP and alternative "physical" diagnoses can be explored simultaneously and this, after all, is the usual paediatric practice of exploring more than one diagnostic option in the early stages of patient assessment. The outcome is affected by delay in diagnosis.

In addition, paediatricians routinely assess the relationship of the child and family as they deal with illness, and this assessment is of particular importance in MSBP.

PROTECTION OF THE CHILD

Once it is clear that MSBP is likely, action to protect the child is essential. In most jurisdictions, professionals are obliged to notify suspicions of child abuse, including MSBP as a form of child abuse, to child welfare/child protection authorities. Separation of the child and parent is usually needed for the child's protection, at least in the short-term. The team responsible for assessing the child should decide who should convey to the family that MSBP is being considered. The circumstances in which this information is passed to the family must be carefully considered. Empathy is required. The parent, even while inflicting suffering on the child, feels pain as a parent. Parents may respond to this information that MSBP is likely, or even suspected, with anger, by inducing fabricated other illnesses "to prove the doctor is wrong", or even by removing the child from the health care institution or to another area. Whether or not separation occurs at this stage, there must be increased vigilance around the time that the diagnosis is communicated to the family. Assessment of the risk to siblings is required urgently. In child abuse, decisions on continuing parental involvement in the care of the child and participation in decision making is always difficult. In MSBP, where lying and denial are central components of parental behaviour, great caution must be exercised when the child is left in the parent's care.

CHILD'S MEDICAL NEEDS

The child will have medical needs which must still be met even if the diagnosis of MSBP is accepted. While there may be no new episodes of induced or fabricated illness, there are often residual effects of previous induced illness, invasive investigations and complications of treatment. Thus, there must be detailed medical plans to reverse many of these effects, whenever possible. For example, when there have been technological interventions, such as a tracheostomy, a gastrostomy or placement of a central line for parenteral nutrition, the need for the intervention must be carefully assessed. Some, or all, may no longer to be needed, but detailed medical supervision is essential as he/she returns to "normal". When presumed allergens have been part of MSBP, then there needs to be a trial of exposure under controlled situations. When there have been induced or fabricated seizures, anti-seizure medication may be reduced carefully, again under close observation. A disease such as asthma may have been grossly over treated with systemic steroids, and these must be reduced slowly, again monitoring for side effects and recurrence of the disease. Issues as apparently simple as the duration of iron supplements in iron-deficiency anaemia need to be considered carefully. Many of the children have permanent scars from the abuse directly, or indirectly from treatment. Such scars, their emotional impact and need for plastic surgery need to be considered in the overall treatment plan.

Children who already have a chronic illness and on whom MSBP is superimposed pose difficult problems. They may be difficult to place in foster care. In general, the paediatrician who already knows the child should follow the child long-term because of the multiplicity of medical concerns, and because of the existing connection with the family and the child.

Whether or not the child has a chronic illness, continuing medical supervision is required. While induced illness and fabrication may cease, these children are still subject to everyday illness and injuries requiring medical care.

PSYCHOSOCIAL ISSUES

The victims most need help in the area of psychological and social functioning. The literature indicates that there are commonly problems in this area, but is less helpful in the specifics of treatment. Children placed in foster homes need a warm, loving and nurturing environment, and this can generally be achieved. For infants, this may be all that is required in the way of treatment. For older children, the objectives of treatment must be developed first, and detailed plans developed in association with child welfare/child protection services. Issues of separation, whether temporary or permanent, needs to be settled early and if children are permanently separated from their parents, attempts should be made to keep siblings together. The existence of phobias, depression and separation anxiety needs to be addressed. Social skills are often deficient and separate and emphatic action is required to correct these. If long-term separation is ordered, appropriate counselling is required to deal with grief and anxiety. Counselling may be provided by many different professionals and professions, such as child psychiatrists, psychologists, social workers, nurse counsellors and so on. In some cases, treatment will be given to the child by supporting and helping the foster parent in their everyday interactions with the child.

A detailed psychosocial assessment is essential, whoever is going to be ultimately responsible for treatment. A child psychiatrist will often be involved to focus on the degree of psychological disturbance of the child and current parent/child interactions. Intensive counselling is required over many years, which may be given by professionals in a number of disciplines. The counselling must be well coordinated as different professionals and different modalities may be used over time. It is not possible to generalise on which modalities will be used, as this will depend on the specific situation. Some examples include behaviour modification, hypnosis, play therapy and group therapy, but in individual cases, many other modalities of treatment may be used. All require that trust develop between the therapist and child.

FAMILY INVOLVEMENT

If the child is returned to the family, close supervision and monitoring by child welfare authorities is essential. This must be long-term. The treatment and support for the parent(s) and family system must be well coordinated with treatment for the child. Coordination of the psychological treatment for the child and family and physical treatment of the child is also required.

While specific counselling will be carried out by psychologists, psychiatrists, social worker or another counsellor, those involved at the time of the original diagnosis have a continuing role. For example, it can be reassuring to the child to have continuity in at least one of the professionals. The team involved in the diagnosis can be helpful in discussing changes in plans and objectives, and then reminding authorities of the reason for the treatment plan in the first place!

OUTCOME

The outcome of MSBP is not known in any detail. There should be no surprise at such a state of affairs, given the difficulties in diagnosis and follow-up. In some ways the literature has more information on the outcome of undiagnosed and unidentified cases, than on proven cases. In proven cases, much of the information and outcome is conditioned by the specific nature of the fabrications, and the professional response to this fabrication by way of investigation and treatment. Thus, all complications of investigations and treatment could be compiled from published literature and considered outcomes of MSBP! The overall outcome is less well known.

MORTALITY

Death is one outcome of MSBP. The precise mortality rate is unclear, and some cases resulting in death appear in more than one report. Ways of establishing mortality rates have varied. Waller (1983) contacted the doctors who had described MSBP and non-accidental poisoning, and found that in the 23 cases he located at least five of the children were known to be dead. Rosenbergh (1987) reviewed the published literature between 1966 and 1987 and calculated a mortality rate of 9%. In a review of 54 MSBP cases deliberately poisoned, Henretig (1995) reported that nine (16.67%) had died. In a report of a more specific form of poisoning, non-accidental salt poisoning, Meadow (1993) reported that of 12 children seen over 15 years, one had died. Alexander et al. (1990), reported the case of two siblings (and five puppies) who died over a short period of time due to arsenic poisoning. Prospective studies are less common, but provide unique information. In one excellent study over two years, McClure et al. (1996), identified 128 children in the United Kingdom, of whom eight (6.24%) died. This study included MSBP from many different classes.

When apnoea or non-accidental suffocation is a feature of MSBP, death is mentioned in a number of reports. Mitchell et al. (1993) reported on 11 children from five families seen over ten years and reported two deaths in this small group. In another series, Alexander et al. (1990) reported

13 children in five families of which apnoea was a dominant feature in three families, and in one of the cases apnoea ceased when the child was placed in a foster home. Further investigations in the families revealed that the previous child with unexplained apnoea who went on to die, and although the death had been labelled "unexplained" it was likely to be homicide/ MSBP. Meadow (1996) described 27 children in which there was suffocation of apnoea, and this group included nine who died. That same report noted that there had been 18 deaths among siblings, most diagnosed as sudden infant death syndrome (SIDS).

OUTCOME FOR SIBLINGS

Considerable information on outcome is available from the detailed report of the investigation of alleged suffocation by parents by Southall *et al.* (1997). This group used covert video surveillance (CVS) in 39 patients suspected of child abuse and in 30 confirmed suffocation and in a further three saw other severe forms of abuse. The 39 patients investigated had 41 siblings of whom 12 had died a sudden and unexpected death. Eleven of these deaths had been diagnosed as SIDS, but subsequently the parents admitted suffocation in the case of eight children (four families). There was evidence of abuse in 15 other living siblings. Despite the association between many cases of MSBP and SIDS, the converse that most cases of SIDS are associated with MSBP or homicide, is untrue. SIDS is a natural phenomenon, and parents whose child dies from this cause deserves support and sympathy. However, the possibility that apnoea was a precursor of SIDS was first raised by Steinschneider in 1972. Following publication of this study, apnoeic episodes were assumed to be a precursor of SIDS. This assumption changed attitudes towards SIDS, the treatment and investigation of apnoea, and research endeavours in SIDS. Steinschneider's report was published before MSBP was recognized, but in the New York Times (1994), it was reported that the mother of the children in the case reports had in fact confessed to suffocating her children. In a review of the related issue of early childhood death, Pitt and Bail (1995) cited 51 articles dealing with the topic (from 115 they had reviewed). Infanticide was noted as dating back to the beginning of recorded history, but this detailed review did not provide information on what leads parents to murder of their children. Reece (1993) provided criteria to distinguish SIDS from fatal child abuse and although the phrase MSBP is not used, the description includes this syndrome.

PHYSICAL SEQUELAE

Of the non-fatal outcomes, only a few will be mentioned. One of particular importance is cerebral damage. This is mentioned in a number of reports. Saulsbury (1984) reported an 11-month-old boy with recurrent apnoea and seizures who had a respiratory arrest due to hydrocarbon pneumonitis, which in turn followed an intravenous injection of an hydrocarbon by the mother. The infant survived but with developmental delay, cortical blindness and cerebral palsy. The mother of one of the cases reported by Alexander *et al.* (1990) when age 17 had "resuscitated" an infant she was babysitting. This infant survived with brain damage. It seems likely that this was a case of MSBP, and one of those many in which a diagnosis was never made, yet sequelae were obvious.

Another outcome worthy of note is progression of pre-existing disease, particularly when there is non-compliance with treatment to such an extent that MSBP is considered likely. Godding and Kruth (1991) in a review of 1648 patients with asthma identified 17 families (18 children) as having MSBP. Eleven of them were undertreated and one died during an episode of severe asthma. Seven were overtreated.

Detailed and systematic follow-up of victims of MSBP gives different information from individual case reports. Such a study was reported by Bools *et al.* in 1993. This group was aware of 100 families in which a child had suffered MSBP. Detailed study was confined to 54 families whose addresses were known, and who could be contacted for follow-up to establish the current status of the child. There were 24 boys and 28 girls, who were grouped by presenting features as follows: smothering (15), poisoning (13), seizures (14), miscellaneous (12). Further fabrications were seen in 30 children who stayed with their mother, across all four groups of original presentations. Adequate data on current status was obtained on 38 of the 54. Twenty-seven had significant disease, in ten there were signs of gradual improvement but 17 showed no evidence of improvement. There were physical concerns due to severe brain injury resulting in developmental delay and quadriplegia (one each). Most of the concerns were behavioural, such as school non-attendance, concentration difficulty, underachieving, and emotional, conduct and behavioural difficulties. It was not possible to decide which specific feature led to a better prognosis, given the range of severity of the initial abuse and lack of standardization of legal procedures. Thus there was a substantial psychological morbidity, but the fact that improvement was seen in some, is reassuring that careful assessment and planned individual management strategies can decrease the risk of long-term difficulties.

PSYCHOLOGICAL OUTCOME

Psychological morbidity was also described in detail in six children (McGuire and Feldman, 1989). Developmentally appropriate behaviour problems were seen, varying from feeding disorders in infants, withdrawal and hyperactivity in pre-school-age children, to hysterical disorders and personal adoption of Munchausen Syndrome behaviour in adolescence. Even when active participation and abuse by the parent ceases or just decreases, there are still significant psychological problems in the child.

Co-morbidity was studied by Bools et al. (1992) in 56 families, and was found in 41 (73%). These problems were failure to thrive (16, 29%), non-accidental injury or neglect (16, 29%) and other fabrications (36, 64%). This group did not deal with emotional abuse because of the difficulty of identification and description in a retrospective study. As mentioned earlier in a large study using covert video surveillance of children with suspected suffocation, Southall et al. (1997) reported other forms of abuse in these children, such as broken legs.

The long-term psychological and physical impact is not clearly known, as many victims are never identified, and others are lost to follow-up as soon as child protection supervision ceases. Libow (1995) examined the childhood experience and long-term psychological outcome for ten adults (33 to 71 years of age). These were all self-identified victims of illness fabrication, and completed a 33-item questionnaire with demographic and open-ended questions, and a check list of psychological symptoms supplemented by telephone interviews. In addition to the emotional and physical problems in childhood, most reported problems in adulthood. These included insecurity, avoidance of medical treatment, and post-traumatic stress symptoms. Most of the siblings had been abused physically or medically. Some expressed considerable residual anger towards abusing mothers. There was a surprising degree of sympathy for the fathers who had passively colluded or failed to protect. Some of the parents involved in MSBP continue to fabricate their own illness and to harass their adult children with fabricated dramas years later. Siblings of patients fare poorly and death has been noted in siblings of index cases in a number of studies cited earlier in the chapter. The morbidity of siblings has been specifically studied (Bools *et al.*, 1992). Of 56 patients, 44 (43%) had suffered from child abuse, 40 (39%) were victims of MSBP and 18 (17%) had failure to thrive, non-accidental injury, were neglected or given inappropriate indications. Eleven (11%) had died with the cause of death being medically inconclusive. These high morbidity and mortality figures are likely to be under reported as full data was not available on 20%, some were at decreased risk of abuse as they were not living with the mother, or under protection from child welfare services.

A detailed personal account has been published under the title "My mother caused my illness: The story of a survivor of Munchausen by Proxy Syndrome" (Bryk and Siegel, 1997). This adult chronicles her experience as a child through eight years of abuse, in traumatic and harrowing terms. Her hospital record as a child indicated 28 hospitalisations, 24 surgeries, multiple blood transfusions, dozens of X-rays, numerous incision and drainage procedures and skin and bone grafts. These followed episodes of medical abuse with the earliest memories between the ages of two and three. The mother restrained the child, was very angry, and hit her legs with a hammer. The fractures and infections required extensive medical treatment. Eventually the child stood up to the mother and told her she was going to tell the teacher and the doctor, and the mother at this stage ceased to abuse this child. The medical condition improved dramatically, and the child had the full use of her legs for the first time in eight years. There were several subsequent corrective surgeries but the worse was over for her. The sibling then became the target. Still, many years later, there is great hurt that the father did not believe or protect his child. The mother continues to be a liar and a deceptive actress, causing long-term and continuing pain to this survivor.

CONCLUSION

There is clear evidence that there is significant morbidity and mortality if MSBP is not diagnosed, and significant physical and psychological morbidity and mortality even if diagnosed. Thus, management demands early diagnosis, and planned individual treatment and long-term counselling for the child, and at the same time specific treatment for the family.

REFERENCES

Alexander, R., Smith, W., Stevenson, W. (1990). Serial Munchausen Syndrome by Proxy. *Pediatrics* **86**: 581–585.

Bools, C. N., Neale, B. A., Meadow, S. R. (1992). Co-morbidity associated with fabricated illness (Munchausen Syndrome by Proxy). *Arch. Dis. Child.* **67**: 77–70.

Bools, C. N., Neale, B. A., Meadow, S. R. (1993). Follow-up of victims of fabricated illness (Munchausen Syndrome by Proxy). *Arch. Dis. Child.* **69**: 625–630.

Bryk, M., Siegel, P. T. (1997). My mother caused by illness: The story of a survivor of Munchausen's by Proxy Syndrome. *Paediatrics* **100**: 1–7.

Emminson, D. M., Postlethwaite, R. J. (1992). Factitious illness: Recognition and management. *Arch. Dis. Child.* **67**: 1510–1516.

Godding, V., Kruth, M. (1991). Compliance with treatment in asthma and Munchausen Syndrome by Proxy. *Arch. Dis. Child.* **66**: 956–960.

Henretig, F. (1995). *The Deliberately Poisoned Child in Munchausen Syndrome by Proxy*, eds. Levin, A.V. and Sheridan, M. S. (Lexington Books, New York).

McClure, R. J., Davis, P. M., Meadow, S. R., Sibert, J. R. (1996). Epidemiology of Munchausen Syndrome by Proxy, non-accidental poisoning & non-accidental suffocation. *Arch. Dis. Child.* **75**1: 57–61.

McGuire, T. L., Feldman, K. W. (1987). Psychologic morbidity of children subjected to Munchausen Syndrome by Proxy. *Pediatrics* **83**: 289–292.

Meadow, R. (1993). Non-accidental salt poisoning. *Arch. Dis. Child.* **68**: 448–452.

Meadow, R. (1990). Suffocation, recurrent apnoea, and sudden infant death. *J Pediatr* **117**: 351–357.

Mitchell, I., Brummitt, J., DeForest, J., Fisher, G. (1993). Apnea and factitious illness (Munchausen Syndrome) by Proxy. *Pediatrics* **92**: 810–814.

New York Times, March 25, 1994.

Reece, R. M. (1993). Fatal child abuse and sudden infant death syndrome: A critical diagnostic decision. *Paediatrics* **91**: 423–429.

Rosenbergh, D. A. (1987). Web of deceit: A literature review of Munchausen Syndrome by Proxy. *Child Abuse Negl.* **11**: 547–563.

Saulsbury, F. T., Chonbanian, M. C., Wilson, W. G. (1984). Child abuse: Parental hydrocarbon administration. *Pediatrics* **73**: 719–722.

Southall, D. P., *et al.* (1997). Covert video recordings of life-threatening child abuse: Lessons for child protection. *Pediatrics* **100**: 735–760.

Steinschneider, A. (1972). Prolonged apnea and the sudden infant death syndrome: Clinical and laboratory investigations. *Pediatrics* **50**: 646–654.

CHAPTER 15

Ethical and Public Policy Issues in the Management of Munchausen's Syndrome by Proxy (MSBP)

GWEN ADSHEAD

Honorary Senior Lecturer/Consultant in Forensic Psychotherapy, Broadmoor Hospital, St George's Hospital Medical School and Traumatic Stress Clinic, Middlesex Hospital

Ethics in medicine and child abuse are both topics that generate passionate emotions. The study of bioethics particularly addresses those dilemmas which occur when clinicians interact intimately with vulnerable people, who are dependent on them. Doctor–patient relationships are simultaneously similar to, and different from, relationships between parents and children; but both types of relationship involve discrepancies of power, and the potential for abuse of that power. Perhaps for these reasons, the state retains an interest in both doctor–patient and parent–child relationships.

Munchausen's Syndrome by Proxy (MSBP), and its management, raises a number of different ethical dilemmas, which arise in the context of both doctor–patient, and parent–child relationships. In this chapter, I will argue that many of these dilemmas arise because clinicians are involved in different relationships simultaneously, which give rise to conflicting duties. This produces anxiety in clinicians, which may be expressed as denial, as anger or in clinical decisions which are later regretted. I will look at the different relationships involved; the duties they entail, and the nature of the conflicts engendered. I will then endeavour to put these interpersonal conflicts in a wider social context, and address the urgent question of the doctor's duty vis-à-vis society; whether doctors have ethical duties as citizens which are no less strong than their professional ethical duties.

DOCTORS, PATIENTS AND DUTIES

Traditionally, the doctor and the patient form a relationship when the patient initiates contact, seeking help from the doctor. The doctor is understood to be a competent carer who can provide help to the patient who is both needy, and not able to supply his own needs. In this sense, the patient is dependent on the doctor, who is able to exert power over the patient, not only by virtue of the patient's dependence, but also in terms of the doctor's superior knowledge base.

This power discrepancy is tempered by the doctor's professional duties to the patient, that is, to treat her not only with professional competence, but also with respect. This respect includes not only the requirement to obtain consent from the patient before action, but also to keep information about the patient private. The power discrepancy is also tempered by the trust which develops between the doctor and the patient. Philosophers (such as Whiteley, 1969) have argued that duties are a function of a trust relationship. The ground of any duty is always a specific feature of the situation; in this case, the trust relationship between the professional and some other person or persons.

The doctors' duties are formalised both in professional ethical codes for doctors, and in relevant case law and statutes. Both legal jurisdictions, and professional regulatory bodies, acknowledge the importance of the doctor–patient relationship, and especially the trust which is part of that relationship. A dependent relationship, with such a power differential, can only be successful if both parties can trust one another. Legal and ethical safeguards are not a substitute for the establishment of trust, and most doctors (and indeed nurses) are trained to see their relationships with individual patients as imposing an over-riding set of duties upon them.

However, this ideal vision of the doctor–patient relationship "trumping" all other concerns is in reality not so easy to maintain. Doctors are subject to other duties apart from those due to their patients. For example, doctors must obey the criminal law; a doctor will not be excused criminal responsibility on the grounds that their criminal act assisted their therapeutic relationship, as the debate about euthanasia demonstrates. Doctor–patient relationships are to some degree regulated by various civil laws, that is, doctors must not act negligently, and are bound by legislation relating to public health, such as the registration of some diseases. Doctors are not outside the body politic, and may have duties as citizens which may conflict with their professional duties; as a counterexample, most doctors are excused jury service (a civic duty) because of their clinical commitments. Finally, doctors may have personal duties to their families, friends and themselves; even if they frequently ignore these duties, this does not mean they do not exist.

There are also professional specialities where the doctor–patient relationship does not consist solely of two people. Public health physicians have duties to communities, ranging from small to very large. Such doctors may find their duties of a much more civic and political nature. Many general practitioners would argue that when they are involved with multiple members of one family it is hard to keep a tight boundary between the relationships, since the health of one affects the health of the rest, both mental and physical. This is especially true of the health of children, whose identity is developing, and for many years is embedded in their relationships with their parents and siblings. It is arguably not possible to have a professional relationship with an individual child patient, because of their dependence on their primary carers. The most obvious example of this is on the field of obstetrics, where mother and child are at one level indistinguishable. In general paediatrics, most practitioners recognise the importance of involving the carers of a child in its care; not least because for many years, the carer will not only have to speak for the child, but be the agent of the treatment.

Although children can be patients (in terms of making autonomous decisions in conjunction with a doctor), most sick children have only minimal autonomy, which is embedded and facilitated by their relationships with their caretakers. Therefore, the paediatrician finds herself involved not in one doctor-patient relationship, but a set of relationships, which may be best seen as overlapping circles.

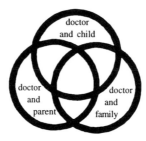

Fig. 1.   Doctor and child, doctor and parent, doctor and family.

Figure 1 describes only the inter-personal relationships relating to the individual child patient. However, as suggested above, doctors are involved in other relationships beyond the one with the patient; so there are further circles to add:

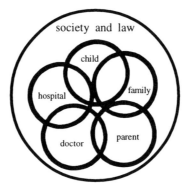

Fig. 2.   Three original circles plus, doctor and the rest of the hospital, doctor and the law.

The doctor's dilemma is exacerbated by uncertainty about:

  the nature of her duties to each party
  the scope of her duty to each party
  whether the nature of the duties to each party are different and
    if so, how
  whether all duties are equally weighted
  what to do when those duties conflict

THE CASE OF MSBP

How does this analysis apply in the case of the paediatrician involved in a case where MSBP is suspected? It may be helpful to distinguish decision making before and after clinical suspicion is alerted. Since most cases involve non-speaking children (i.e., usually under three), the paediatrician is certainly going to be involved both with the parent and the child. Before suspicions are raised, the doctor will relate principally to the parents; often the mother as the most common primary carer. What is not so clear is whether the mother is the main beneficiary of the doctor's professional duties. As I have suggested above, even though the paediatrician may have some ethical and legal duties to the mother, they may be out-weighed by the doctor's duties to the child. Further, as Southall (1997) has suggested, the doctor's duties to the mother may only exist insofar as they assist the mother (and the doctor) to take care of the child. This would be consistent with English law on consent to medical treatment, whereby parents can consent for the child if, and only if, the treatment is on the child's interests. Parents cannot consent to procedures which do not benefit the child. This scenario of course is relevant in those cases of factitious disorder where the parent(s) either insist on multiple investigations, or cause those investigations to be done unnecessarily.

Nevertheless, the paediatrician's initial relationship will be with the parent and the child, and the doctor will rely on the therapeutic relationship with the parent in order to provide best care for the child. Let us consider now what happens to the doctor–patient relationship when the clinicians suspect MSBP as a cause of the child's symptoms. As suggested by Emminson (this volume) and others, trust is an essential part of the doctor–patient relationship, especially in paediatrics. Most doctors assume that their patients (including the mothers of patients) are telling the truth. This assumption is a feature of nearly all public–professional relationships, and should not be taken as a sign of credulity. The assumption that people are not telling the truth is usually confined to certain very specific professional groups, or situations: police investigators, interrogators, war or some business situations. In such situations, the professionals have very different relationships with the subjects with whom they are involved; policemen do not have clients, let alone patients. Very few doctors would see themselves as being in any way similar to police interrogators.

There is another important therapeutic aspect to the assumption of truth. Assumptions about whether a person is telling the truth are also judgements about that person's honesty; and doctors are repeatedly instructed during their training to be non-judgmental, as a way of building up a therapeutic relationship. A non-judgmental stance is both a reflection of medicine's scientific status (i.e., science is value neutral) but also a statement about medicine's essentially benevolent nature. Of course, this notion of medicine being non-judgmental is a myth, but a very important one professionally, and doctors are therefore reluctant to give it up.

This means that doctors and nurses working with MSBP parents will, at some point, find themselves deceived. The issue of deception and deceit is clearly an important dynamic factor in MSBP; it seems likely that one of the main reasons that MSBP generates so much emotion is that deceiving health care professionals is a key feature of the behaviour. Given the importance of deception to the MSBP parent, it is not surprising that health care professionals and child protection agencies should also find themselves using deception themselves. This is most obvious in relation to the use of covert video surveillance in hospitals to detect MSBP behaviour. The use of such a system has caused enormous ethical disquiet and debate (Foreman and Farsides, 1993; Gillon, 1995; Southall and Samuels, 1996; Shinebourne, 1996; Thomas, 1996). The disquiet arise from two aspects of the procedure; first that given that there is a suspicion of child abuse, to leave the child with the parent is treating the child like a "tethered goat". Second, the suspected parents are not told that they are under suspicion, but are allowed to believe that they and their child are being treated just as normal within a hospital. In actuality, the suspected parent(s) is the subject of police investigation, under the auspices of child protection legislation. Thus the therapeutic relationship, (and the hospital setting in which it takes place), becomes more like the relationship between police and criminals in which no party can be trusted, and suspected criminals may be invited to entrap themselves unwittingly.

For the paediatric doctors and nurses, this change from therapeutic process to the criminal justice process, represents a loss of trust which is distressing for the staff, and ultimately for the MSBP parent. Especially, doctors and nurses can no longer see themselves as non-judgmental, and impartial in the face of adversity. Using hospital premises and therapeutic procedures to detect a criminal is a challenge to the ideal of medicine to which most health care professionals aspire. What is ironic is that the use of covert video in this way is a repetition of the deception that MSBP parents use to gain the doctor's attention, that is, they rely on the trusting nature of the therapeutic agents involved in the medical process to carry out their behaviour. Just as both parent–child and doctor–patient relationships are based on trust, MSBP appears to be a betrayal of the child's trust, which is expressed in a further breakdown of trust between doctor and parent.

MEDICAL ETHICS, PUBLIC POLICY AND CHILDREN

There are many areas of conceptual muddle in an ethical analysis of MSBP, and the response of doctors. First, although it is common for doctors to talk about "diagnosing MSBP", in fact MSBP is a behaviour. It is not yet established as either a disease or an illness. There is some evidence to suggest that not all so-called MSBP behaviours are the same; what is known is that a considerable proportion of such behaviours closely resemble the intentional physical abuse of children (Donald and Jureidini, 1996). The intentional infliction of harm to a child is (at least potentially in most jurisdictions) a crime. What many paediatric teams are therefore faced with is the suspected commission of a crime on their professional premises, where the victim is the object of a professional duty of care, and the suspected perpetrator is the principal carer for that object.

Legally, there can be little doubt about the nature and scope of a doctor's duty here. The doctor has a duty of care to the child, which would certainly include the prevention of any *medical* harm. It is debatable whether there is any duty to prevent *any* harm; however, given the vulnerability of the child, and the fact that most MSBP children are detected as inpatients, it is quite possible that a court would conclude that hospitals had a duty of care to prevent harm to child inpatients. Such a duty would be likely to include preventing possible harm from their parents. Child protection legislation exists to protect children who are at risk, and although doctors are not bound by that legislation, good medical practice requires that they cooperate with child protection proceedings (Department of Health, 1991).

It is in the ethical realm that the dilemmas caused by MSBP still seem so painful. It seems to be counter to every ethical ideal of medicine to use the therapeutic relationship to entrap people; even if they are suspected of child abuse. These are suspects who are not cautioned, but who are allowed/encouraged to think that they are safe in hospital. Many paediatricians want to call such parents "patients", even if the formal duty of care between them is limited. Most paediatricians are also aware that the vast majority of such parents are damaged and disabled people who are in need of medical psychiatric help. If a hospital is a place for healing, how could it be that one could go there, and end up arrested and charged with a serious offence?

The counter arguments must run as follows. First, given that doctor–patient relationships rely on trust, that trust has been betrayed by the parent who lies to the clinical team. It is hard to think that a doctor's relationships with a patient who lies, and with a patient who tells the truth, are morally equivalent. This does not, of course, mean that the doctor has carte blanche to treat badly any patient who lies; only that the ethical nature of the relationship, and its application may be different.

Second, although paediatricians have some duties to parents of sick children, it seems hard to argue that the primary object of the duty of care is not the child, or that parents' needs should outweigh the child's need for protection. Even if the parent is in some sense the patient of the paediatrician, on behalf of the child, they are not a patient in quite the same way as the child who is ill; nor can they remain a patient in this limited sense where there appears to be good grounds for suspecting the parent of abusing the child. There are other health care professionals who can take responsibility for the health needs of the parent; there is no one else to take the place of the paediatrician to address the child's needs.

Third, and most painfully, doctors, nurses and hospitals are not outside the law. If an alleged crime is taking place on hospital premises, then all health care professionals, as citizens, have an interest in stopping that crime.

The more difficult question is whether there is a professional duty to prevent crime, that is, a duty that develops during a specific training, and which is imposed on the completion of that training, based on the acquisition of a specialist knowledge. This seems more difficult to argue. Some clinicians (e.g., Shepherd, 1995) hold the view that doctors should take active steps to prevent violence; especially given the specific professional costs to the National Health Service. Arguably, since most doctors are contracted to work for the NHS, all doctors have a professional duty to reduce costs. One obvious difficulty is that the training in medicine does not provide any of the specific training that is normally required for crime detection, investigation and resolution. Professionals who have had such a specific training are usually called policemen. By virtue of this training, they are awarded special powers by the state in pursuit of their professional task, which is the protection of public safety. These special powers include the power in certain circumstances to invade people's privacy and freedom, and limit their liberty.

Confusion may arise because on completion of their training, doctors are also given special powers, which include the invasion of normal privacy, and access to specialised information about people. But it seems obvious that this is for an entirely different purpose. The police are given statutory powers (carefully regulated) for the protection of the public as a whole; doctors are awarded professional privileges, which are not nearly so carefully regulated, (certainly not by statute) in order to better the health of the patients to whom they offer care. This distinction is crucial to the argument about covert video surveillance in MSBP. It is the police who investigate the suspected crime of child abuse, and not the doctors, who have no public mandate to do so, nor the requisite training. Confirming the occurrence of a crime is not the same as diagnosis; not least because it has implications for the suspect's place in society which are quite different to those which follow the diagnosis of an illness.

Finally, it is of some interest to consider that there is a strong tradition within medical ethics for doctors to deceive in order to benefit the patient; most commonly in those situations where doctors have not told patients the truth about their condition to prevent them distress. In the past, this question was one of the commonest dilemmas raised in bioethics (Bok, 1979; Jackson, 1991), and doctors have argued strongly for the professional right to deceive in order to do good. The difference between that situation and MSBP is that the doctor's deception may well do the child physical good; may even save the child's life. However, the child is not deceived; and for the person who is actually deceived, the doctor's deception may have adverse consequences.

CONCLUSION

Doctors are part of a wider society, as is the criminal justice process. It is not possible ethically or legally for a clinician to argue that their therapeutic relationships take them outside a social domain in which all citizens have an interest. Therefore, doctors should have no concern that they are acting unethically when they are acting to protect children from crime, even if the alleged perpetrator is also known to the doctor therapeutically. However, there is equally no duty on doctors to act as accessory policemen. In fact, there is real danger if they do so, that doctors will not be able to then fulfil their duty to act justly, which is important for all members of the medical profession; both professionally and as citizens.

REFERENCES

Bok, S. (1979). *Lying*, Vintage Books, New York.
Department of Health (1991). Working together: Guidelines in the management of suspected child abuse. London.
Donald, T., Jureidini, J. (1996). Munchausen's Syndrome by Proxy. Child abuse in the medical system. *Arch. Paediatr. Adoles. Med.* **150**: 753–758.
Foreman, D., Farsides, C. (1993). Ethical use of covert videoing techniques in detecting Munchausen Syndrome by Proxy. *Br. Med. J.* **307**: 611–613.
Gillon, R. (1995). Covert video surveillance by doctors for life threatening Munchausen's Syndrome by Proxy. *J. Med. Ethics* **21**: 131–132.
Jackson, J. (1991). Telling the truth. *J. Med. Ethics* **17**: 5–9.
Shinebourne, E. (1996). Covert video surveillance and the principle of double effect: A response to criticism. *J. Med. Ethics* **22**: 26–28.

Southall, D., Samuels, M. (1996). Guidelines for the multiagency management of patients suspected or at risk of suffering from life threatening abuse resulting in cyanotic-apnoic episodes. *J. Med. Ethics* **22**: 16–21.

Southall, D. (1997). Covert video recordings of life threatening child abuse: Lessons for child protection. *Paediatrics* **160**: 735–760.

Shepherd, J., *et al.* (1995). Should doctors be more proactive as advocates for victims of violence. *Br. Med. J.* **311**: 1617–1621.

Thomas, T. (1996). Covert video surveillance — an assessment of the the Staffordshire protocol. *J. Med. Ethics* **22**: 22–25.

Whiteley, C. H. (1969). On duties. In Feinberg, J. (ed.). *Moral Concepts.* Oxford University Press. pp. 53–60.

CHAPTER 16

Current Challenges in the Management of Perpetrators

DEBORAH BROOKE

Consultant Forensic Psychiatrist,
Bracton Centre, Bexley Hospital, Kent

GWEN ADSHEAD

Honorary Senior Lecturer/Consultant in Forensic Psychotherapy,
Broadmoor Hospital, St George's Hospital Medical School and
Traumatic Stress Clinic, Middlesex Hospital

> Deception occupies a central and privileged place in forensic psychiatry.
>
> (Gunn *et al.*, 1993)

Psychiatrists generally have limited experience of those who induce or fabricate illness in children. There are two reasons for this. Firstly, these behaviours are rare. McClure *et al.* (1996) examined the epidemiology of MSBP, non-accidental poisoning and non-accidental suffocation. They found an annual incidence of 0.5/100,000 children aged under 16 years, "an incidence approximately equal to death from drowning in children under 16 or cystinosis in the under five-year age group". Secondly, perpetrators tend to use somatic mechanisms to contain distress, rather than, for example, seeking help for anxiety or depression. Thus, they may shun psychiatrists, and have frequent attendances at other clinics. This chapter has been written in the hope that interest in these perpetrators by psychiatrists can be increased, and research stimulated, so that the knowledge base of psychiatry, and forensic psychiatry in particular, may be increased.

DIFFICULTIES IN ASSESSMENT

The assessment of an alleged perpetrator of MSBP has differences from many other assessments in psychiatry. Firstly, a note on the setting. If you are seeing someone in the context of court proceedings, expect them to be overwhelmingly distressed at the loss of their child. The gender of the interviewer may affect the dynamics of the interaction; perhaps, if possible, such perpetrators should not be interviewed by obviously pregnant psychiatrists. It is difficult to assess a condition characterised by secrecy and deception in one single interview. The usual "one-off" interview and report may not do justice to the interpersonal difficulties exhibited by perpetrators. In this respect, these individuals resemble those with severe personality disorder. One should expect a lengthy period of evaluation.

When assessing people who are accused of interpersonal violence, it is necessary to pay as much attention to personal relationships as to the individual themselves.

There may be evidence in the history of long-standing difficulties in social, occupational and emotional relationships. The full picture may not emerge unless several informants are interviewed.

Detailed information should be elicited about the subject's views of her pregnancies, the planning or otherwise of pregnancies and her experiences of pregnancy and labour. Ask about the family of origin, because of Welldon's view (see Chapter 4) that the perversion of mothering spans three generations. Lastly, Griffith (1988) remarked on the importance of the dynamics of the mother's *partner's* family, too. He described two families in which the mother — perpetrator, already exhibiting a somatoform disorder, joined a nonassertive partner from an enmeshed, authoritarian family system with a history of exploitation of children.

Early developmental experiences of the perpetrator are crucial to understanding the pathology of the parent-child relationship, which will subsequently be manifest in MSBP behaviour in its various forms. Particularly important aspects of the history are:

- a family tree including a description of the physical and mental health of any parental figures

- childhood experiences, including the history of significant attachment figures, any child abuse, chronic childhood illness and experiences of loss
- does the subject remember being frightened as a child, and of whom?
- clues to the development of self esteem, including relationships with peers from early schooldays
- adolescence is a crucial time for the expression of personality difficulties, as evinced by the development of delinquency, substance misuse and sexual activity
- details of the past medical and psychiatric history, including deliberate self-harm. Are they a frequent attender at surgeries and clinics? Is there evidence of factitious disorder or somatoform disorder?
- expectations and views of the parenting role, and of the child or children

The assessment of these individuals may be complicated by denial. This is a common finding among child abusers (Salter, 1988). Feldman (1994) has commented upon the pervasive denial of responsibility among perpetrators, even when confronted with compelling evidence. Denial may reflect a lack of empathy, a psychological strategy in the face of adversity, or legal advice pre-conviction. Doctors may expect their patients to give a full account of themselves, but this is not to be expected in the assessment of alleged perpetrators. Failure to disclose may indicate deception, but may also reflect a profound inability to trust others. Given that histories of childhood deprivation and abuse are common in such perpetrators (Bools *et al.*, 1994), it is not surprising that they find it hard to trust. Day (Parnell and Day, 1998) describes the importance of the development of trust within the therapeutic relationship, enabling the perpetrator to acknowledge her abusive behaviour. This may take many months. During this time, a fuller history of abuse and difficulties experienced by the perpetrator may emerge, confirming the inadequacy of a single assessment interview.

There are no standardised instruments that will assist us in assessing interpersonal difficulties in these individuals. Most psychological instruments focus on the psychopathology of the individual, rather than their relationships. Most tools for rating parent–child interaction were designed for less pathological groups. Even hospital notes reflect this bias. Perpetrator's notes only tell us about the individual; paediatric notes only tell us about the child.

DIAGNOSIS

Because these peoples' difficulties are intrapersonal, as well as interpersonal, established diagnostic labels do not convey the full extent of their problems. Studies of psychiatric status of perpetrators (Samuels *et al.*, 1992; Bools *et al.*, 1994; Southall, 1997) report frequent histories of abuse, self-harm, factitious or somatisation disorder and substance misuse. Bools *et al.* (1994) described the findings at a standardised psychiatric interview with 19 perpetrators, only two of whom were not given a diagnosis. Half of them had psychiatric symptoms, such as fatigue and somatic symptoms. Three subjects were given a "mental illness" diagnosis, as follows: eating disorder, hypochondriasis, probable recent psychosis, and 17 were given personality disorder diagnoses.

DEFINITION OF PERSONALITY DISORDER

Personality disorders are defined as "a severe disturbance in the character-ological constitution and behavioural tendencies of the individual, usually involving several areas of personality, and nearly always associated with considerable personal and social disruption" (ICD-10; World Health Organization, 1992). The multiaxial classification used in DSM-IV (American Psychiatric Association, 1994) has the particular advantage of emphasising both acute symptomatology (diagnosed on axis 1) and concomitant personality disorders (diagnosed on axis 2). Further axes allow a reference to other important conditions, such as psychosocial and environmental problems. The multiaxial system facilitates comprehensive and systematic evaluation.

DIFFICULTIES WITH THIS CONCEPT

Current classifications of personality disorder have limitations. Women commonly do not meet the behavioural criteria for antisocial personality disorder, the diagnosis of which is heavily influenced by criminal activity. In women, interpersonal criteria are more relevant than offending behaviour. If these are considered, the diagnosis of antisocial personality disorder is less likely to be missed (Hare, 1998). There may be omissions from current classifications. Bass and Murphy (1995) have argued strongly that disorders characterised by multiple, recurrent and frequently changing unexplained physical symptoms (somatisation disorder in ICD-10, somatoform disorder in DSM-IV), currently conceptualised as a mental illness, should be regarded as a personality disorder because of the youthful age of onset, the enduring nature of the syndrome and the finding that two thirds of these individuals meet criteria for other personality disorders. They argue that somatoform disorders, as well as personality disorders, should be seen as disorders of development.

The label "personality disorder" has been regarded as unhelpful. It can be used to exclude a patient from treatment (Lewis and Appleby, 1988), and psychiatrists may therefore have less experience in treating such patients. Concomitant states of anxiety and depression may be missed entirely. The label does not provide information about prognosis or risk.

There remains much work to be done in elucidation of the connection between various features of personality disorder and the disordered behaviours that cause concern. We lack information about the prognosis and best management for different degrees of personality disorder. This simple diagnostic label gives only the most basic level of information about a patient. This poses real difficulties for professionals, especially in the area of risk assessment.

PROBLEMS WITH LEGAL AND PSYCHIATRIC OUTCOMES

Psychiatrists may be asked to assess these patients in connection with care proceedings, in which fitness to parent, and/or the risk of significant harm to the child in the future, may be key questions. Adult psychiatrists cannot usually claim expertise in the assessment of parenting, which is generally carried out by child psychiatrists.

In the United Kingdom, the majority of inducing or fabricating mothers who are convicted of injuring their child receive a probation order, possibly with psychiatric treatment, either voluntarily or mandated by the court ("probation with a condition of treatment"). Small numbers receive a prison sentence, or in-patient treatment in a specialised facility, such as the Cassell Hospital, and some are managed under the Mental Health Act, 1983 (MHA). Of this last group, those with the legal category of mental illness (those who, for example, had a depression underlying their behaviour towards the child on the background of some personality strengths) might be expected to be managed within general psychiatric services. Those with a diagnosis of personality disorder are placed in the legal category of psychopathic disorder. They are doubly disadvantaged, combining the two groups for which forensic psychiatric services are the least developed: women and the personality disordered. Medium secure services have extreme difficulty in providing a safe therapeutic environment for women patients because they are greatly outnumbered by men (Maden, 1997) and those with emotionally unstable or antisocial personality disorders have largely been excluded from general psychiatry services (Cawthra and Gibb, 1998). Traditional "medical model" psychiatric units have, generally, only limited success in treating personality disorder. This model encourages dependency which, counter-productively, elicits hostility from many such patients. Thus, if a perpetrator with psychopathic disorder is thought to meet the "treatability" (or, prevention of deterioration) criteria in the Mental Health Act, she is most likely to be treated in one of the maximum secure ("special") mental hospitals (Broadmoor, Park Lane or Rampton) because of the limited alternatives in medium security, plus the length of time and the specialised expertise required to treat severe personality disturbance.

Thus, the disposals available to the psychiatrist range from those with, potentially little impact on the patient to those with, inevitably, enormous impact. Are they justifiable differences, or do they reflect our lack of therapeutic options for people whose offending clearly has psychodynamic origins?

While the special hospitals offer substantial opportunities for rehabilitation and therapy within a safe and containing environment, there are disadvantages. Detention in special hospital is a deeply constraining and stigmatising experience (Warner, 1996). The removal of patients to distant institutions, with attendant difficulties in maintaining community links, is contrary to current thinking in the organisation of services for mentally disordered offenders (Home Office, 1992). It is a major deficit in forensic services that treatment options for women with severe personality disorders are so limited.

The position is even more bleak for male perpetrators. The available evidence suggests that men who offend against children in their care are dealt with more severely than women, even for offences of similar seriousness. This is particularly true in cases of infanticide, the killing of a baby under one year (Marks and Kumar, 1993). Possible reasons for this general finding are explored by Wilcynski (1997). She sums up the impact of gender on sentencing in cases of child homicide as "filicidal women are more likely to be actually mentally ill than filicidal men; they are also more likely to be labelled as mentally ill". The result is that a larger proportion of male perpetrators receive a prison sentence.

CONCLUSIONS

While it is a truism to write that research is needed, it is difficult to offer services in the absence of an evidence-based strategy. The necessary evidence is likely to be provided by research done with different populations in different ways. For example, we need more information about the exact nature of the difficulties faced by these parents in looking after a dependent child. What is it about dependency and vulnerability that seems to arouse such a disturbed response in these individuals? A better understanding of their early childhood experiences may help us to understand their relationships with their own children; and may, coincidentally, throw some light on the causation of the interpersonal difficulties with characterise personality disorder. Research may need to be done across disciplines and involve both children and parents. Long-term follow-up studies of children and perpetrator parents would assist us in making good quality prognoses.

There is still further research to do upon the efficacy of different interventions for personality disorder, to establish the best ways to help people who are clearly damaged.

The various personality disorders discussed here are thought to have childhood adversity as an aetiological factor. In some families, the damage starts in earliest infancy. Repairing or even containing these degrees of damage is a lengthy and demanding endeavour, posing a challenge, not only to psychiatry, but to all social structures.

REFERENCES

American Psychiatric Association (1994). *Diagnostic and Statistical Manual, Fourth Edition.* APA, Washington, DC.

Bass, C., Murphy, M. (1995). *J. Psychosom. Res.* **39**: 403–427.

Bools, C., Neale, B., Meadow, R. (1994). *Child Abuse Negl.* **18**: 773–788.

Cawthra, R., Gibb, R. (1998). *Br. J. Psychiatry* **173**: 8–10.

Feldman, M. (1994). *Int. J. Psychiatry Med.* **24**: 121–128.

Griffith, J. (1988). *Fam. Process* **27**: 423–437.

Gunn *et al.* (1993). Deception, self-deception and dissociation. In: *Forensic Psychiatry, Clinical, Legal and Ethical Issues* (Butterworth Heinemann, Oxford) p. 407.

McClure, R., Davis, P., Meadow, S., Sibert, J. (1996). *Arch. Dis. Child.* **75(1)**: 57–61.

Hare, R. (1998). *Legal and Criminological Psychiatry* **3**: 99–119.

Home Office. *Review of Health and Social Services for Mentally Disordered Offenders and Others Requiring Similar Services.* HMSO, London, 1992, Final Summary Report, p. 7.

Lewis, G., Appleby, L. (1988). *Br. J. Psychiatry* **153**: 44–49.

Maden, A. (1997). *International Review of Psychiatry* **9**: 243–248.

Marks, M., Kumar, R. (1993). *Med. Sci. Law* **33**: 329–339.

McClure, R., Davis, P., Meadow, S., Sibert, J. (1996). *Arch. Dis. Child.* **75**: 57–61.

Parnell, T., Day, D. (1998). *Munchausen Syndrome by Proxy: Misunderstood Child Abuse* (Sage Publications, Thousand Oaks, California) pp. 167–182.

Salter, A. (1988). *Treatment of Child Sex Offenders and Their Victims* (Sage Publications, Newbury Park, California).

Samuels, M., *et al.* (1992). *Arch. Dis. Child.* **67**: 162–170.

Southall, D., *et al.* (1997). *Paediatrics* **100**: 735–760.

Warner, S. (1996). In: *Special Women? The Experience of Women in the Special Hospital System*, ed. Hemingway, C. (Avebury, Ashgate Publishing Ltd., Aldershot) p. 60.

Wilcynski, A. (1997). *Child Homicide* (Greenwich Medical Media Ltd. London) pp. 117–146.

World Health Organization (1992). *The ICD-10 Classification of Mental and Behavioural Disorders* (WHO, Geneva).

CHAPTER 17

New Directions in Research and Service Development

CHRISTOPHER BOOLS
Consultant Child, Adolescent and Family Psychiatrist,
Child & Family Therapy Service,
St Aldhelm's Hospital Frome

INTRODUCTION

Before considering possible research and developments for the future, I wish to take an overview of what is already known about MSBP. Whilst studying this book, two things may have struck the reader. Firstly, there are many published accounts of single examples of MSBP although only a small number of case series reported. Secondly, whilst there is usually plenty of paediatric detail, there are relatively few accounts presenting psychiatric detail of the fabricator, or emotional and behavioural information about the child.

There are two outstanding issues concerning MSBP. Firstly, the problems of terminology which will facilitate multidimensional classification in both paediatric and psychiatric systems. Secondly, the effects of intervention with important implications for the continuing development of services, notably the roles of social agencies with statutory responsibilities for child protection and health services "Working Together" (Home Office *et al.*, 1991). Very few accounts report the response of the fabricator to treatment and subsequent development of the child victims. These latter areas are the most difficult to study, perhaps for a combination of reasons; the rarity of MSBP, the nature of MSBP itself, and the necessary follow through period to report meaningfully on outcome. However, a useful amount is known about the individual psychopathology and family interactions at the time of the presentation of the index MSBP abuse. There are few detailed accounts of events preceding the fabrications with the notable exception of a detailed narrative account (Loader and Kelly, 1996).

A further critical issue is the process of education and training of professionals in health services, social services and the legal profession (Ostfield and Feldman, 1997; Williams, 1986) all of whom provide services for MSBP victims, fabricators and their families. This process began relatively recently and is ongoing. One can envisage a similar process to that which followed the recognition of physical abuse and later sexual abuse of children, and the changes in practice which followed in the three professional areas (health, social services and legal); these have all amounted to sea changes. The emotional impact on health services staff has been reported (Blix and Brack, 1988) and may have a very significant impact on management. As has been discussed in an earlier chapter, the response to being deceived is a particular issue for health services staff. I suspect that we have some way to go in being able to provide the optimum opportunities for treatment with rapid access to appropriate resources sometimes presenting a challenge. A well co-ordinated management and treatment programme for MSBP will consume potentially a large quantity of limited resources, often requiring specialist facilities which may not be available locally.

THE PROBLEM OF TERMINOLOGY

Earlier in the book there has been discussion on the confusion regarding the use of terminology, notably to what, or whom, the term Munchausen Syndrome by Proxy refers. To try to help clarify the use of terminology (and the boundaries of MSBP) the American Professional Society on the Abuse of Children (APSAC) created a task force which reported in 1998 (Ayoub and Alexander, 1998). Perhaps the main problem with terminology has been the use of the term Munchausen Syndrome by Proxy to refer to three elements of the fabricating situation, these are; the process of the fabrication, victimization of the child, and a psychiatric disorder of the parent. Each of these elements or dimensions of the MSBP "scenario" requires classification to which I will return below.

In order to clarify thinking and the use of terminology, APSAC recommend that;

1) **Pediatric Condition** (illness, impairment, or symptom) **Falsification (PCF)** is a form of child maltreatment in which an adult falsifies physical and/or psychological signs in a victim, causing the victim to be regarded as ill or impaired by others. It is a subgroup of the larger **Abuse by Condition Falsification** category of victimization in which the victim is another individual, adult or child. A child who is subjected to this behaviour is a victim of **PCF** and should be coded as such using the DSM-IV with the additional opportunity to state if the abuse is physical, emotional or combined type. Note that PCF can occur in the absence of FDP, for example, a parent who injures a child and lies about the circumstances, or children who present with illness or conditions resulting in school non-attendance where the parent motivation is to keep the child at home — the child is likely to collude.

2) The fabricator/perpetrator has the psychiatric diagnosis of **Factitious Disorder by Proxy** (FDP). The fabricator intentionally falsifies the history, signs or symptoms in the child to meet their own self serving psychological needs. In the DSM-IV (American Psychiatric Association, 1994) the code would be Factitious Disorder Not Otherwise Specified (300.19). There are, however, more specific proposed criteria in the section of the DSM-IV "criteria sets and axes provided for further study" called "research criteria for factitious disorder by proxy".

These proposals helpfully separate the process of fabrication from (one of) the possible psychiatric diagnosis(es) applicable to the perpetrator. It could be debated whether fabricating behaviour of this type should receive a psychiatric diagnosis. For example, other varieties of deceptive behaviour (Sheridan, 1995) such as fraud and imposturing would not. Furthermore the question of motivation (one of the APSAC proposed criteria) is complex and is considered later in this chapter.

The APSAC proposals allow for separate recording of the type of abuse of the child. There is then the potential for further development of the classification with a focus on the impact on the child. For example, the classification of abuse could be recorded using the system developed by Crittenden (Claussen and Crittenden, 1991). Emotional abuse could be further defined, possibly based on the scheme developed by Glaser in the United Kingdom (Glaser, 1995), and an attempt made to grade severity. This would be of great practical value if combined with developmental and psychiatric assessments of the child and a formulation of the broader mother child relationship. Broad categories of disturbance in the parent child relationship may be useful for research and legal purposes (Sturge, 1998).

The approach taken by the editors in a forthcoming book (Eminson and Postlethwaite, 2000) is to use the term Munchausen Syndrome by Proxy Abuse (MSBP abuse) to refer to the process of what happens to the child. Although they are not recommending the same terminology, both APSAC and these British workers are taking the same approach, that is, to separate the term for what happens to the child from a psychiatric diagnosis of the fabricator. It is interesting that APSAC are recommending losing the term MSP or MSBP which may not be easy to achieve.

What is the way forward with terminology? Firstly, it would be helpful to develop a process to reach a consensus in the United Kingdom. Recommendations could then be made which would parallel those made by APSAC in the United States of America. It would then be possible for the appropriate contributors of the ICD (World Health Organization, 1992) and the DSM-IV to consider further how their respective classifications will be organised. At the present, the ICD is less specific than the DSM-IV as there are no specific categories for either the fabricator or the victim — the victim is categorised in a cover all group (T74.8) as a victim of child abuse.

SUBTYPES OF FABRICATION

To allow more specific classification, the method of fabrication may be divided into three broad operational subtypes which has been previously suggested (Bools, 1996). This would be compatible with the approaches taken by APSAC (they would be subtypes of PCF) and Eminson and Postlethwaite. An outline of the suggested subtypes is;

1. Verbal fabrication.
2. Verbal fabrications plus the falsification of specimens or charts.
3. Fabrication associated with production of physical signs (by smothering, poisoning, withholding nutrients and medicines and other means).

The production of physical signs could also be called "Illness Induction Syndrome", although unfortunately there is potential for some confusion as this term was used for all the subtypes in the Great Ormond Street study (Gray and Bentovim, 1996).

In addition, and complementary, to the above subtypes I had also suggested considering other aspects of the fabrication in three "special situations";

  i. fabrication of psychiatric disorder,
 ii. factitious disorders in pregnancy and,
iii. fabrication in the presence of genuine physical illness.

LIMITATIONS OF PUBLISHED RESEARCH

The nature and rarity of MSBP have placed restrictions on the methods of research that have been possible in a number of key ways;

1. There have been only a small number of studies of case series reported. The four largest I will refer to as the Leeds group (Bools, Neale and Meadow, 1992; 1993; 1994), the Great Ormond Street group (Gray and Bentovim, 1996; Gray, Bentovim and Milla, 1995), the Brompton/Staffordshire group (Samuels, McLaughlin et al., 1992) and the Leeds/Cardiff epidemiological group (McClure, Davis, Meadow and Silbert, 1996; Davis, McClure et al., 1998)
2. Within series, many factors to be accounted for have been heterogeneous:
   a. the nature of the fabrications
   b. the consequent variety and severity of physical and emotional abuse
   c. the psychopathology of the perpetrators, often with incomplete psychiatric diagnoses

d. the family situations and support available to the fabricator
e. the additional care and support available to the child victim
f. the intervention
g. the follow through period, which usually has not been very long

It may be useful to consider some of the various strengths and weaknesses of these series. In the Leeds group, the range of fabrications was very wide. The follow-up was reasonably long for a number of children, however, the group was heterogeneous with a wide range, both of the ages of children at follow-up and the duration of follow-up. With regard to fabricating mothers, not all were interviewed, although those that were provided a good level of information utilising standard research instruments. When combined with case note data this was likely to lead to reasonable accuracy of psychiatric diagnosis. Most of the interviews with mothers were carried out some time after the fabrications had been discovered so the psychopathology would have had time to change. The range of interventions following discovery was very wide from no specific intervention to adoption with no contact. It is important to note that some of fabrications had been carried out some years before the study commenced.

The particular strengths of the Great Ormond Street series are that all the cases had been seen at the one hospital over a defined period. This meant that there were more details gathered about the fabrications and psychiatric matters at that time. In addition, the initial interventions were less heterogeneous than those in the Leeds group study since they were carried out by staff at the hospital and later by locally based professionals after close liaison with hospital staff. Although it was possible to report in detail on some aspects of the psychiatric histories of fabricators, a weakness was that there was no standard assessment of the mental state or personality of the fabricators. The nature of the fabrications was again somewhat heterogeneous with ten cases of active with-holding of food, five alleged allergy with insufficient food, 15 alleged serious illnesses and 11 actively harmed. The follow through interval was also short.

In the series reported by the Brompton/Staffordshire group, the abuse by upper airways obstruction, was the same in every case resulting in the most uniform of the reported series. From the psychiatric perspective there was comprehensive data collection by discusion with the 14 psychiatrists who saw the mothers shortly after the discovery of the fabrications in order to reach consensus about diagnosis, combined with information from general practice records and social service records. However, a relative weakness is that the 14 mothers were not interviewed by a single investigator and no standardised instruments were used to record the psychiatric status.

The study of the largest series, and with the best methodology from the epidemiological point of view, has been by the combined Leeds and Cardiff team. (Note that there were 128 cases of MSBP combined with non-accidental poisoning and non-accidental suffocation over two years across the United Kingdom and the Republic of Ireland. Calculation resulted in rates of combined annual incidence of 0.5/100,00 in children under 16 years and 2.8/100,00 for children under one year). The level of concern was standardised with each case requiring a child protection case conference to be held. Psychiatry was not the focus of the study and from this perspective the study lacked detail. There was no standardised assessment of the emotional and behavioural state of the children or psychiatric status of the fabricators by the research team. An excellent feature of the study was the rate of follow-up, although the interval was only 24 months. However, I offer a caution; although the re-abuse rate included three cases of emotional abuse, the children were not directly assessed and the likelihood of under identification of subsequent abuse, including abuse of siblings and more subtle forms of emotional abuse is suggested.

APPROACHES TO FURTHER RESEARCH

These large (and expensive) studies illustrate many of the difficulties encountered in producing findings to assist clinical practice. Is the best way forward to attempt a large (macro) study as suggested by Runyan (Runyan, 1998) below? This would require a large number of cases in a series. Alternatively, are other approaches likely to produce more useful findings. There could be small (micro) studies looking at qualitative aspects in single cases or small numbers.

The first issue for any new study will be reporting of cases using an agreed set of criteria and terminology, which results in a classification with sufficient multidimensional detail to be clinically meaningful. There should be good descriptions of interventions used and the response of the fabricator, with a reasonably long follow-up period. In the United Kingdom, prevalence has been well reported and what is now needed urgently is more on prognosis.

PROSPECTS FOR A MACRO STUDY

Because MSBP is a rare problem, in order to collect sufficient cases for the statistical implications of any findings to be meaningful any study will require multi-centre co-operation. The Leeds Cardiff epidemiology study used this method with the assistance of the British Paediatric Surveillance Unit. Early advice from a statistician and use of the power statistic (Sackett, Haynes, Gunyatt and Tugwell, 1991) will determine how many subjects are required to allow the demonstration of a particular difference. In order to gather together a sufficient number of subjects the centres could be spread across national boundaries. Otherwise in order to collect say 150 cases from only the United Kindom and Ireland the study would need to continue for two to three years (based on the Leeds Cardiff annual incidence data).

Many of the issues arising from such a potential study were recently presented by Runyan (1998). When studying rare diseases, the preferred method is a case control study. Identifying a particular control group is a particular issue for MSBP, for example, the next child seen by the paediatrician with a disorder of the same system could serve as a control for each MSBP case.

The ethical difficulties would be specially problematic in a prospective study of MSBP, with the most problematic issues being the refusal to participate and subsequent partial and low overall rate of participation of invited families. Drop-outs are particularly harmful to the overall validity of the study. A further issue is the specific nature of untreated MSBP fabricator currently believed to present a high risk of later abuses which would have to be reported to the appropriate agencies if discovered. A problem similar to this also occurs in a follow-up study when families previously lost to follow-up are re-discovered.

Despite these difficulties potentially affecting any study of child maltreatment which follows through abused children, two large multi-centre projects are underway. LONGSCAN involves the collaboration of investigators at five sites across the United States of America which all have identical study definitions, coding, instrumentation and data entry (Runyan, Curtis and Hunter *et al.*, 1998). A second study, WorldSAFE, is beginning in at least four countries for which the core protocol took four years to develop (Runyan, 1998). These studies benefit from modern technology of e-mail and web sites for data collection. In the United Kingdom, the study reported as "Development After Physical Abuse in Early Childhood" (Gibbons, Gallagher, Bell and Gordon, 1995) is an account of the methods and results of a follow-up of 170 abused children. The reader is directed to the book in which the breadth of assessment is detailed. Although neither of these studies involve MSBP they do illustrate what is possible with planning and long-term committment.

ASSESSING THE RESPONSE TO INTERVENTION

In order to allow standardisation of assessment and the specifics of intervention, it is desirable that subjects pass through one centre where treatment interventions are carried out. The response to intervention is the key practice issue for psychiatrists. The study carried out at The Park Hospital, Oxford (Berg and Jones, 1999), reports the outcome of children whose families had been admitted to The Park Hospital for intensive assessment and treatment by an inpatient based multidisciplinary psychiatric team. Information prior to publication is that 17 children and their families are reported on with a follow-up period of an average of 27 months. The Park study is unique because of the highly specialised nature of the inpatient facility which almost certainly represents the most intensive resource available in the United Kingdom able to admit the whole family, that is, two parents as well as the children.

PROSPECTS FOR PROSPECTIVE "MICRO" STUDIES

"Micro" studies could look at more detail in individual or small numbers of cases in which detailed description of psychopatholgy and processes is valuable. Whether studies are large or small, the use of standardised rating instruments is recommended (Ferguson and Tyrer, 1989). In addition, researchers could draw upon qualitative research methods from the social sciences (Mason, 1998). It would be helpful, and inform clinical practice, to report in detail of the process of change during treatment, particularly noting changes in the mental state of the fabricator and any effects on the child in the short to medium term.

PARTICULAR ISSUES

The central problem of deception in MSBP may limit the value of direct observation of the fabricator's behaviour, and the usefulness of research and clinical methods on which they rely. Information from an informant which can be utilised by a research instrument, such as in the assessment of personality using the Personality Assessment Schedule (Tyrer, 1988), will be invaluable.

The value of personal report by the victim may be the most valid way of finally judging the outcome for children, possibly taking their view at adolescence or into adulthood (Bryk and Siegel, 1997).

INVESTIGATION OF PSYCHOPATHOLOGY

In the clinical setting, the psychiatric formulation will be applied to each individual fabricator for its clinical value as discussed in Chapter 12. Some aspects of the formulation, such as psychological defence mechanisms, are extremely difficult, or impossible, to investigate in an empirical manner. However, it may be possible to investigate particular aspects of the clinical formulation, for example, specific or general learning difficulties, are easily investigated with the use of commonly used standard instruments. Attachment difficulties are a topic of growing interest. For example, the Parental Bonding

Instrument (Parker, 1983) used in our own research, although unpublished, produced interesting findings with regard to the fabricating mothers perception of their own mothers. Both feelings of inadequate care and idealisation of care were reported.

I have drawn attention to the critical issue of motivation with regard to the APSAC criteria for PCF. Motivation for an action is usually a very difficult issue to investigate. This will be especially so for a set of behaviours that involve deception, and when child protection procedures are ongoing and possibly also criminal proceedings. When the death of a child has occurred, whether or not the situation is suspected MSBP, the question of motivation will have legal implications. Even in this situation, it has still been possible to construct a classfication of filicide with motivation as a critical issue (Wilczynski, 1997). It may be that a more accurate account of motivation will become available many years after fabrications are identified which was the case whilst carrying out our own study (Bools, Neale and Meadow, 1994). Nevertheless, early on an attempt to look at motivation should be made. One possible method would be to separate belief from action in the first instance. For example, fabricating mothers have been described, and encountered by myself, who seemed to believe that their child was afflicted by an undiagnosed illness. The fabrication could then be seen in part to result from misperception of ordinary physiology based on this false belief and, ultimately, an attempt to convince a doctor that something is really wrong. The strength of the belief may be an overvalued idea (McKenna, 1984), or less likely a delusion, and both the personality of the misperceiver and the social context will be important considerations. Qualitative descriptions which are integrated with theoretical approaches to aid explanation are also helpful (Loader and Kelly, 1996; Black and Hollis, 1996).

A further issue regarding the assessment of motivation, as part of the overall assessment of dangerousness, is the intent. It has been suggested that intent to harm is not directly related to the actual behaviour carried out and the harm resulting in the child, that is, that a very medically dangerous act may be associated with less intent to harm than a less medically dangerous act. Furthermore, intent may change from moment to moment. Impulsiveness is in itself an important consideration and a further source of potential dangerousness by contrast with planned behaviours.

EFFECT OF INTERVENTION ON OUTCOME

It would be helpful if some of the features of cases of MSBP in which a good outcome has been achieved were reported with respect to the specifics of intervention. In particular, details of the timing and the nature of professional interventions would be helpful and the opinions of clinical workers as to when important changes have occurred would be interesting.

Detail of possible study of legal interventions is beyond the scope of this chapter. However, from a clinical perspective, the benefits for the child of working with a family in the short-term and moving to long-term therapeutic work, combined with social work supervision, with or without a court order, are important practical situations to be examined.

DEVELOPMENTS OF CLINICAL SERVICES

Roles of Professionals

The active co-operation of adult psychiatric services with child & family psychiatric services is likely to be one way forward. For example, in Oxford a detailed personality assessment is carried out by adult psychiatry colleagues, whilst families are being assessed and treated at the family inpatient unit. One of the difficulties for clinicians is the range of psychopathology in terms of severity (and by implication changeability) as well as qualitative diversity. The implication is that clinicians will need to be familiar with a wide range of treatment facilities from outpatient care to secure environment.

The Importance of Feedback to Professionals

The concern expressed about the implementation of "care plans" by local authorities with a suggested "audit of implementation" by the court (Thorpe, Lord Justice and Clarke, 1998) over perhaps two years could bring forth new opportunities for data gathering in a multidisciplinary environment and ultimately improved lives for children and their parents.

REFERENCES

American Psychiatric Association. (1994). *Diagnostic and Statistical Manual of Mental Disorders*, 4th edition, APA.

Ayoub, C., Alexander, R. for APSAC Munchausen by Proxy Task Force. (1998). Definitional issues in Munchausen by Proxy. The APSAC Advisor **11**: 7–10.

Berg, B., Jones, D. PH. (1999). Outcome of intervention in Factitious Illness by Proxy. *Arch. Dis. Child.* **81**: 465–472.

Black, D., Hollis, P. (1996). Treatment of a case of Factitious Illness by Proxy. *Clin. Child Psychol. Psychiatry* **1**: 89–98.

Blix, S., Brack, G. (1988). The effects of a suspected Munchausen's Syndrome by Proxy on a pediatric nursing staff. *Gen. Hosp. Psychiatry* **10**: 402–409.

Bools, C. N., Neale, B., Meadow, S. R. (1992). Co-morbidity associated with fabricated illness (Munchausen Syndrome by Proxy). *Arch. Dis. Child.* **67**: 77–79.

Bools, C. N., Neale, B., Meadow, S. R. (1993). Follow-up of victims of fabricated illness (MSBP). *Arch. Dis. Child.* **69**: 625–630.

Bools, C. N., Neale, B., Meadow, S. R. (1994). Munchausen Syndrome by Proxy: A study of psychopathology. *Child Abuse Negl.* **18**: 773–788.

Bools, C. (1996). Factitious Illness by Proxy: Munchausen Syndrome by Proxy. *B. J. Psychiatry* **169**: 268–275.

Bryk, M., Siegel, P. (1997). My mother caused my illness: The story of a survivor of Munchausen by Proxy Syndrome. *Pediatrics* **100**: 1–7.

Claussen, A. H., Crittenden, P. M. (1991). Physical and psychological maltreatment: Relations among types of maltreatment. *Child Abuse Negl.* **15**: 5–18.

Davis, P., McClure, R. J., Rolfe, K., Chessman, N., Pearson, S., Sibert, J. R., Meadow, R. (1998). Procedures, placement, and risks of further abuse after Munchausen Syndrome by Proxy, non-accidental poisoning and suffocation. *Arch. Dis. Child.* **78**: 217–221.

Eminson, M. E., Postlethwaite, R. J. (2000). *Munchausen Syndrome by Proxy: Fabricated illness in Children* (Butterworth-Heinemann, Oxford).

Ferguson, B., Tyrer, P. (1989). Rating instruments in psychiatric research. In: *Research Methods in Psychiatry: A Beginner's Guide*. eds. Freeman, C. and Tyrer, P. (Gaskell, London).

Gibbons, J., Gallagher, B., Bell, C., Gordon, D. (1995). Development after Physical Abuse in Early Childhood. HMSO.

Glaser, D. (1995). Emotionally abusive experiences. In: *Assessment of Parenting: Psychiatric and Psychological Contributions* eds. Reder, P. and Lucey, C. (Routledge, London).

Gray, J., Bentovim, A., Milla, P. (1995). The treatment of children and their families where induced illness has been identified. In: *Trust Betrayed; Munchausen Syndrome by Proxy, Interagency Child Protection and Partnership with Families* eds. Horwath, J. and Lawson, B. (National Children's Bureau, London) 149–162.

Gray, J., Bentovim, A. (1996). Illness induction syndrome; paper 1 — a series of 41 children from 37 families identified at Great Ormond Street Hospital for Children. *Child Abuse Negl.* **20**: 655–673.

Home Office *et al.* (1991). Working Together Under the Children Act, 1989. HMSO.

Loader, P., Kelly, C. (1996). Munchausen Syndrome by Proxy: A narrative approach to explanation. *Clin. Child Psychol. Psychiatry* **3**: 353–363.

Mason, J. (1998). *Qualitative Researching* (Sage Publications, London).

McClure, R. J., Davis, P. M., Meadow, S. R., Sibert, J. R. (1996). Epidemiology of Munchausen Syndrome by Proxy, non-accidental poisoning, and non-accidental suffocation. *Arch. Dis. Child.* **75**: 57–61.

McKenna, P. J. (1984). Disorders with over-valued ideas. *B. J. Psychiatry* **145**: 579–585.

Ostfeld, B. M., Feldman, M. D. (1997). Factitious disorder by proxy: Awareness among mental health practitioners. *Gen. Hosp. Psychiatry* **18**: 113–116.

Parker, G. (1983). *Parental Overprotection: A Risk Factor in Psychosocial Development* (Grune & Stratton, London).

Runyan, D. (1998). Defining the epidemiology of Munchausen Syndrome by Proxy: The case for collaborative studies. Presented at Stockholm conference, August 1–2.

Runyan, D., Curtis, P., Hunter *et al.* (1998). LONGSCAN: A consortium for longitudinal studies of maltreatment and the life curse of children. *Aggression Violent Behav.* **3**: 245–255.

Sackett, D. L., Haynes, R. B., Guyatt, G. H., Tugwell, P. (1991). Deciding on the best therapy. In: *Clinical Epidemiology: A Basic Science for Clinical Medicine* Second Edition, Chapter 7. (Little Brown, Boston).

Samuels, M. P., McLaughlin, W., Jacobson, R. R., Poets, C. F., Southall, D. P. (1992). Fourteen cases of upper airways obstruction. *Arch. Dis. Child.* **67**: 162–170.

Sheridan, M. S. (1995). Deception in society, and professional proxy and other analogs. In: *Munchausen Syndrome by Proxy: Issues in Diagnosis and Treatment* eds. Sheridan, M. S. and Levin, A. V. (Lexington, New York).

Sturge, C. (1998). Medical input to care planning: The contribution of the child and adolescent mental health services to the care planning process. In: *Divided Duties: Care Planning for Children within the Family Justice System* eds. Rt. Hon Lord Justice Thorpe and Clarke, E. (Family Law).

Thorpe, Lork Justice, Clarke, E. (eds.) (1998). *Divided Duties: Care Planning for Children within the Family Justice System* (Family Law).

Tyrer, P. (1988). *Personality Disorders. Diagnosis, Management and Treatment* (Wright, Bristol).

Williams, C. (1986). Munchausen Syndrome by Proxy: A bizarre form of child abuse. *Fam. Law* **16**: 32–34.

Wilczynski, A. (1997). *Child Homicide* (Greenwich Medical Media, London).

World Health Organization. (1992). *The ICD-10 Classification of Mental and Behavioural Disorders. Clinical Descriptions and Diagnostic Guidelines* (WHO, Geneva).

Index